INTERNATIONAL DEVELOPMENT IN FOCUS

# Human Resources for Mental Health Service Delivery in Viet Nam

## Toward Achieving Universal Health Coverage

SANG MINH LE, ERIC HAHN, TU ANH TRAN, SELIN MAVITUNA, AND TAM MINH THI TA

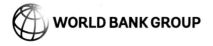
**WORLD BANK GROUP**

# Contents

## Box

## Figures

## Maps

## Tables

# Acknowledgments

This report was prepared by a joint World Bank–German Agency for International Cooperation (GIZ) team led by Sang Minh Le (senior health specialist at the World Bank and author) and consisting of Eric Hahn (deputy program director of GIZ's Hospital Partnerships, head of Global Mental Health at Charité, and author), Tu Anh Tran (consultant at the World Bank and author), Selin Mavituna (psychologist at Charité and author), and Tam Minh Thi Ta (mental health advisor for GIZ's Hospital Partnerships, senior consultant psychiatrist at Charité, and author). Significant contributions were made by Tuyet Minh Bui (consultant), Thang Thi Mai (consultant), and Trang Thi Nguyen (consultant). The Department of Psychiatry at Hanoi Medical University, led by Associate Professor Tuan Van Nguyen, conducted the surveys, workshops, and group discussions that served as inputs for the final report.

The report was prepared under the overall guidance of Aparnaa Somanathan and Ronald Mutasa (practice managers in the World Bank's East Asia and Pacific region, Health, Nutrition and Population Global Practice), Carolyn Turk (country director, World Bank Viet Nam Country Office), and Christophe Lemiere (practice leader, World Bank Viet Nam Country Office). The authors are grateful to peer reviewers Sheila Dutta (senior health specialist, World Bank), Kate Mandeville (senior health specialist, World Bank), Ana Mercado (senior health specialist, World Bank), and Ilhame Ouansafi (health specialist, World Bank), for providing constructive comments on an earlier version of the report. The team thanks Nga Thi Anh Hoang (program assistant, World Bank) for excellent administrative support throughout the preparation of the report. The team also thanks the Viet Nam Ministry of Health; the Viet Nam Psychiatric Association; and the university faculties, psychiatric hospitals, and development partners who participated in meetings, group discussions, and consultative workshops.

The team gratefully acknowledges technical collaboration with Charité Universitätsmediz in Berlin, Germany, under GIZ's Hospital Partnerships program, as well as generous funding from the Japan Policy and Human Resource Development Fund.

# About the Authors

**Eric Hahn** is a medical doctor, consultant psychiatrist, and psychotherapist. He also works as an associate professor and researcher in global mental health and psychotic disorders at Charité – Universitätsmedizin Berlin. In addition to his academic career, he serves as deputy director of the Hospital Partnerships program of the German Agency for International Cooperation (GIZ). The program is funded by the German Ministry for Economic Cooperation and Development, operated by GIZ, and aimed at enhancing health capacities and exchange with nations in the Global South. Over the past 15 years, he has fostered collaboration between Germany and Viet Nam, bolstering mental health infrastructure and expertise in the latter. Recognized for his contributions, he holds an honorary professorship in psychiatry from Hanoi Medical University. His research focuses on genetic psychiatry, attitudes toward psychiatry in low- and middle-income countries, and global mental health, with strong participant- and user-oriented perspectives.

**Sang Minh Le** is a senior health specialist in the World Bank's Viet Nam Country Office, where he works on human resource development in the health sector, digital health, environmental health, and public-private partnerships for health. For 20 years, he has provided policy advice and technical assistance to government agencies and health institutions in Cambodia, the Lao People's Democratic Republic, Myanmar, and Viet Nam. Before joining the World Bank, he worked as a lecturer for a university and as a health expert for a consulting firm based in Hanoi, Viet Nam. He has published several books and numerous study reports. He holds a degree in general medicine, a master's degree in public health, and a diploma in hospital management.

**Selin Mavituna** is a research associate at the Charité – Universitätsmedizin Berlin. With a background in psychology and international relations, she is part of the Global Mental Health Research Group. She is currently contributing to international development cooperation projects funded by the German Ministry for Economic Cooperation and Development that aim to strengthen mental health care in Viet Nam. Her research areas include mental health–related stigma and discrimination, migrant and refugee mental health, and mental health of the LGBTQIA+ community.

**Tam Minh Thi Ta** is a professor of psychiatry and psychotherapy at Charité – Universitätsmedizin Berlin. She supervises psychotherapy for Vietnamese migrants as a senior consultant psychiatrist and trauma therapist. Notably, she established Europe's first university mental health outpatient clinic for Vietnamese-speaking migrants. She aims to establish university mental health cooperation programs between Germany, international research ventures, and collaboration partners in Viet Nam. She holds an honorary professorship in psychiatry from Hanoi Medical University. Her research focuses on Vietnamese migrant mental health and therapeutic knowledge dissemination to enhance Viet Nam's mental health capacities. Her interests encompass women's and children's mental health, migrant mental health, culturally and linguistically tailored psychotherapy, and mental health capacity training in Viet Nam.

**Tu Anh Tran** is a researcher at the National Institute of Hygiene and Epidemiology in Hanoi, Viet Nam. Specializing in data management and analysis, his work mainly focuses on compiling diverse data sets from various sources into comprehensive reports that are used to inform national policy decisions. His expertise extends to collaborating with numerous stakeholders across different levels and sectors of Viet Nam's health care system. During the COVID-19 pandemic, he contributed significantly as a member of the Rapid Response Information Team within the National Steering Committee for COVID-19 Response. He holds a master's degree in public health and a PhD in preventive medicine.

# Executive Summary

## INTRODUCTION

Mental illness is a public health challenge in Viet Nam. It has been estimated that around 15 percent of the Vietnamese population has at least one of the 10 most common mental disorders. People with mental illnesses still have limited access to quality mental health services. The most significant barriers to accessing mental health care in rural areas are the limited availability of health professionals and lack of access to treatment services. Although national health programs have been implemented at the grassroots level, treatment services are limited to people with severe psychiatric and neurological illnesses, including schizophrenia, chronic epilepsy, and drug addiction. Out-of-pocket payments are a significant issue for those with uncovered conditions. The social support network may reach only 30 percent of the targeted population. Due to stigmatization and discrimination, individuals who exhibit mental disorders and their family members seek care and support from informal systems rather than formal ones. The COVID-19 pandemic exacerbated the mental health crisis due to an increase in mental disorders and disrupted critical mental health services.

This report is based on a study that was conducted in response to repeated calls for further actions that address mental health, including research as part of policy advocacy efforts. The study's objectives were to (a) understand the coverage of mental health service delivery, (b) assess the current status of the mental health workforce, (c) describe the constraints to mental health education and training, and (d) propose strategic priorities for transforming the mental health workforce. The report combines rich qualitative and quantitative information from online surveys, focus group discussions, workshops, and a literature review. The report aims to inform the decision-making of the government of Viet Nam on transforming the mental health workforce toward achieving universal health coverage.

## MENTAL HEALTH SERVICE COVERAGE IN VIET NAM

The share of the population covered by mental health services in Viet Nam has improved through four interconnected domains: health care, social welfare, education, and informal systems. The number of psychiatric beds in hospitals and social protection centers has increased. Viet Nam currently has 48 psychiatric hospitals and 28 general hospitals with a department of psychiatry or psychiatric ward, providing nearly 10.5 psychiatric patient beds per 100,000 population in the health care domain. The social protection network, including 31 psychiatric rehabilitation centers and more than 70 general social protection centers, provides care for 15,800 individuals with severe mental illnesses, covering nearly 5 percent of all persons with severe mental illnesses requiring social support assistance.

Although institutional care remains dominant, community-based mental health programs have been implemented. In 2000, the Ministry of Health launched a community mental health program, starting with schizophrenia, expanding to chronic epilepsy, and recently providing services for those with depression or drug addiction. At present, more than 11,100 commune health stations in all 63 provinces deliver essential mental health services, including mental disorder recognition, basic psychiatric treatment, and relapse prevention at the community level. Since 2011, the social sector has implemented a national program on community-based rehabilitation and social assistance for people with mental disorders. The first phase (2011–20) created a foundation for community-based service delivery. The second phase (2021–30) continues to develop more inclusive and comprehensive treatments for individuals with severe mental illnesses or depression and children with autism spectrum disorders. The education sector has made progress in addressing the mental health needs of children and adolescents by introducing inclusive education policies and setting guidelines for school-based mental health services. In addition to formal care, informal mental health services are available and vital for providing care to people with mental disorders. Furthermore, the growth of social networks and online communities has led to the rise of peer support groups.

Despite recent improvements, the mental health systems in Viet Nam still face systematic problems and structural challenges. The uneven distribution of resources for psychiatry leads to unequal access to services across provinces and an urban-rural divide. While the top five cities and provinces have more than 20 psychiatric hospital beds per 100,000 population, the five bottom provinces have less than 1 bed per 100,000 population. Access to institution-based social care and support remains limited in the disadvantaged regions, given the unequal distribution of social protection centers and psychiatric rehabilitation centers across provinces. In particular, the Central Highlands region has only 3.5 psychiatric hospital beds per 100,000 population (threefold lower than the national average) and no psychiatric rehabilitation facility.

The quality of mental health care is a major concern. The dominance of traditional treatment regimens in many psychiatric hospitals restricts the adoption of an evidence-based combination of nonpharmacological interventions, like psychotherapies and psychosocial rehabilitation. The shortage of resources hinders mental health care service providers from reaching and maintaining the required quality of care to meet the basic needs of people with mental disorders and help them toward recovery. Although the government has gradually transitioned to community-based care, various obstacles need to be addressed. The commune health stations are incapable of delivering integrated and comprehensive mental health services beyond the provision and revision of pharmacological treatment for patients with schizophrenia and chronic epilepsy. Except for demonstration models in a dozen locations, most social welfare institutions have inadequate capacity to deliver services for people with mental disorders in their communities. Schools and teachers encounter many difficulties in the inclusive education of students with mental disorders and the implementation of school-based mental health interventions.

## MENTAL HEALTH WORKFORCE IN VIET NAM

Viet Nam has a growing and young psychiatric workforce. The number of psychiatrists more than doubled from 286 to 609 between 2004 and 2021, while the ratio of psychiatrists per 100,000 population increased from 0.35 to 0.62. Mental health care facilities in Viet Nam also employ 557 mental health doctors, who are medical doctors with fewer than two years of postgraduate training in psychiatry. An estimated 1.2 percent of all medical doctors in the country have selected a career in psychiatry. The mental health nursing workforce is also growing—there were three mental health nurses per 100,000 population as of 2020. Currently, the country has a young psychiatric workforce, in which 72.6 percent of the psychiatrists and mental health doctors are younger than 50, and over 75 percent of the mental health nurses are younger than 40.

The psychiatric workforce in Viet Nam is highly urbanized, resulting in disparities in access across geo-economic regions. Almost all the psychiatrists, mental health doctors, and mental health nurses are employed by central- and provincial-level health facilities; therefore, they are concentrated in urban areas with limited outreach services to the rural communities. Even in medium-size and small cities, the recruitment of psychiatrists remains a significant concern. The disparity is evident between cities and provinces in different income groups, ranging from 0.17 psychiatrists per 100,000 population in the 10 lowest-income provinces to 1.13 psychiatrists per 100,000 population in the 10 highest-income cities and provinces. The median number of psychiatrists is 10 times higher in the Red River Delta region (1.14 psychiatrists per 100,000 population) than in the Central Highlands region (0.12 psychiatrists per 100,000 population). Working together with psychiatrists and mental health doctors, the mental health nursing workforce shares the common feature of maldistribution across geo-economic regions.

Psychology has recently been recognized as a formal profession in Viet Nam, and it needs to be better structured in the mental health systems. There are currently only 143 clinical psychologists and psychotherapists in the public health sector, making up a very small proportion (3 percent) of the country's total mental health practitioners. Clinical psychologists and psychotherapists are mainly located in wealthier cities, increasing the urban-rural divide in access to mental health services. Of the 63 provincial health systems, 37 have neither psychologists nor psychotherapists in public health facilities. In the private sector, psychologists and psychotherapists often provide psycho-educational interventions to children with delayed language development, autism, or intellectual disability. School psychology counselors are ill-positioned in the education system as their job description, competency framework, and salary scale have not been regulated.

Although the social service workforce has increased rapidly, the qualification-employment mismatch presents a major challenge to mental health social workers, caregivers, and social collaborators. Among social workers in hospitals and social welfare facilities, 86.5 and 81.5 percent, respectively, have an education degree in a discipline other than social work. Mental health caregivers who provide daily care for people with severe mental illnesses in the social welfare facilities are predominantly women between ages 26 and 45 whose educational attainment is mostly at the undergraduate level in various professions. Most of them reported difficulties in early detection, prevention, and classification of and counseling for mental disorders due to a lack of professional training and tools. At the community level, a hundred thousand social collaborators are participating in a national program on community-based social assistance for people with mental disorders; however, there are policy-level challenges to the sustainable integration of social collaborators into the mental health systems.

Most of the mental health professionals reported that they were only somewhat satisfied with many aspects of their jobs. Fringe benefits, opportunities and rewards, and operating rules and procedures are the three main areas of job dissatisfaction, particularly among young professionals receiving low salaries and those working in large cities.

## MENTAL HEALTH EDUCATION AND TRAINING IN VIET NAM

Career pathways and education frameworks in psychiatry have been established for decades, but quality assurance remains a concern. Only one-third of the medical schools in Viet Nam offer a post-graduate education program in psychiatry, and they supply nearly 100 new psychiatrists per year. The country's education programs are over-prescriptive and not yet fully aligned with competency-based education for psychiatrists. In addition to an out-of-date curriculum, the shortage of resources poses a great challenge to delivering education programs for psychiatry. At almost all the country's medical schools, there are more visiting lecturers than full-time faculty members. Furthermore, the network of affiliated institutions for practice is often overloaded due to too many students from different training programs. Recently, psychiatry faculties have offered certification (nondegree) training courses in response to the increasing demand for continuing medical education. The government has implemented effective policies to encourage and attract people to study psychiatry.

Mental health nursing education and training are insufficient in different ways. The undergraduate nursing curriculum is out of date and not harmonized across educational institutions. Students can take only 2 or 3 credits of mental health classes (including theory and practice) in regular undergraduate nursing programs. In the advanced nursing program, students are trained for up to 6 credits (3 theoretical and 3 practical). Psychiatric nurses are trained at the postgraduate level at only a few nursing schools. Less than 1 percent of mental health nurses receive a certification for continuing medical education.

Thirty-two universities in Viet Nam run an education program in psychology. Most of the programs offer a degree at the bachelor's level, six offer a master's degree, and five offer a doctoral degree. Many educational institutions for psychiatry are concentrated in the Red River Delta and Southeast regions, which creates substantial geographic variation in access to education programs in psychology. Several collaborative programs between Viet Nam and foreign universities have recently been created in clinical psychology. Despite these developments, psychology education in Viet Nam still faces various challenges related to the curriculum and resources for education. The career paths of students in psychology programs often need to be clarified and expanded.

Registration and licensing systems for psychologists, including clinical psychologists, have yet to be established, and this affects graduates' employability and professional promotions.

Education and training for social work include higher education, vocational training, and short-term training. Viet Nam currently has 55 higher education institutions and 21 vocational training institutions for social work, which supply about 6,500 workers to the labor market each year. However, higher education institutions for social work are unevenly distributed across regions. Mental health modules in social work education and training programs are inconsistent. Resources for teaching and learning are limited, especially in specialized areas like mental health. Continuous short-term training programs have been organized regularly for a thousand social workers; however, the programs are insufficient to meet the increasing needs of the social service workforce.

## RECOMMENDATIONS

A national strategic plan should be developed to align mental health workforce development with employer demands and population needs. The relevant stakeholders should work together to analyze the situation, set priorities and targets, and harmonize the supply of and demand for mental health professionals to overcome health system challenges. Special attention should be paid to the systematic problems of the mental health workforce, including the shortage of workers, competency mismatch, skill mix imbalance, maldistribution, and weak workforce governance framework. The purpose is to ensure a sufficient, competent, and well-coordinated mental health workforce toward achieving universal coverage of mental health services.

The development of a sufficient and competent mental health workforce requires substantial changes in the country's education and training systems. Educational institutions for mental health need to balance the criteria for admissions with professional and geographical shortages, develop and adopt competency-based curricula that are responsive to changing needs, expand education programs to a wider scope of professions and degrees, promote interprofessional education to enhance team-based care, strengthen resources for education with an emphasis on faculty development and digital technology adoption, and expand the network of practice sites beyond traditional psychiatric hospitals to outpatient clinics and community-based mental health care settings.

The available mental health workforce should be distributed equitably and sustainably to be fit for purpose and responsive to the most needs. This will require emphasizing the recruitment, deployment, and retention of mental health professionals for disadvantaged provinces, particularly those in the Northern Upland, Central Highlands, and Southwest regions, to close the urban-rural divide in mental health coverage. Mechanisms for the attraction and retention of the health workforce in rural areas should be expanded to the mental health professions. In addition to improving fringe benefits and rewards, more effort should be made to harmonize the operating rules and procedures within mental health facilities. Technology-enabled and collaborative task-shifting and -sharing models should be scaled up to improve access to integrated mental health care in settings with limited resources.

A workforce governance framework is pivotal for creating a conducive environment for mental health professionals. This entails standardization and regulation as well as registration and licensure, particularly in emerging areas such as clinical psychology, school psychology, and social work. The National Medical Council should engage in intensive efforts to realize the legal requirements for licensing examinations for the mental health professions. These activities should be implemented under the leadership of a (self-) governing body that is mandated to set standards for education and practices, keep a register of professionals, and conduct competency examinations for licensure.

Financing is a powerful tool for transforming the mental health workforce toward achieving the goal of universal health coverage. The resource base for the mental health workforce can be developed through investment projects or financial mechanisms, such as the establishment of an innovation fund to strengthen the mental health workforce, expanded public insurance coverage of primary mental health care services, increased incentive packages for skilled professionals in rural areas, and others. Mental health policy makers in Viet Nam should use these financial tools to incentivize mental health providers to integrate mental health care into primary health care and shift from institutional care to community-based care. Special attention should be paid to the attraction and retention of skilled professionals in underserved areas, particularly in the Central Highlands and Northern Upland regions.

# Abbreviations

| | |
|---|---|
| ADHD | attention-deficit/hyperactivity disorder |
| ASD | autism spectrum disorder |
| CDC | Centers for Disease Control (Viet Nam) |
| CHS | commune health station |
| CME | continuing medical education |
| CMHP | community mental health program |
| COVID-19 | coronavirus disease 2019 |
| GIZ | Deutsche Gesellschaft für Internationale Zusammenarbeit (German Agency for International Cooperation) |
| LMICs | low- and middle-income countries |
| SGD | Sustainable Development Goal |
| SMI | serious mental illness |
| SPC | social protection center |
| UHC | universal health coverage |
| VND | Vietnamese dong |

# 1 Introduction

## INCREASED BURDEN OF DISEASE DUE TO MENTAL DISORDERS

Mental illness is a global health challenge. The World Health Organization estimates that mental health problems affect 1 billion people. However, less than 20 percent receive adequate care (WHO 2020b). In conflict-affected settings and low- and middle-income countries (LMICs), the prevalence of mental disorders is estimated to be higher, resulting in an even larger treatment gap (Charlson et al. 2019; Patel et al. 2016). Globally, mental health conditions constitute the most significant burden in terms of disability, accounting for 32.4 percent of all years lived with disability and 13.0 percent of disability-adjusted life years (Bloom et al. 2011; Vigo, Thornicroft, and Atun 2016). Although people living with mental health disorders are at least twice as likely to have additional medical health problems (Otte et al. 2016), individuals with other medical illnesses, such as cardiovascular disease, cancer, or diabetes, have a much higher risk of psychiatric comorbidity (Scott et al. 2016). Overall, untreated and chronic mental illnesses cause earlier mortality of 10 to 20 years, depending on the diagnosis (Walker, McGee, and Druss 2015). The high suicide mortality also accentuates the need for greater coverage of mental health care. Suicide mortality has been estimated at 800,000 deaths per year, or 1.5 percent of all yearly deaths (Fazel and Runeson 2020), disproportionately affecting young people, women, and the elderly in LMICs (WHO 2019a).

Mental disorders limit human development and hinder economic growth. They can impede school attendance and learning, as well as the ability to find a job and be fully productive at work (UNDP 2022). Lost productivity due to two of the most common mental disorders, anxiety and depression, costs the global economy US\$1 trillion each year. In total, poor mental health was estimated to cost the world economy approximately US\$2.5 trillion per year due to poor health and reduced productivity in 2010, a cost that is projected to rise to US\$6 trillion by 2030 (Bloom et al. 2011; *Lancet Global Health* 2020).

Nationally representative studies that were conducted 20 years ago estimated that around 15 percent of the Vietnamese population had at least one of the 10 most common mental disorders (Cuong 2017; Vuong et al. 2011). In line with prevalence estimates of mental disorders in LMICs (Steel et al. 2014), more recent population-based surveys in selected provinces have reported that 14.4 to 20.0 percent of the participants had a clinically significant symptom of one or more of the most common mental disorders (Nguyen et al. 2019; Richardson et al. 2010). The most prevalent mental disorders among Vietnamese adults are substance abuse, with a prevalence of 4 to 5 percent of the population; depression, 2.8 percent; anxiety, 2.6 percent; and (narrowly defined) schizophrenia, 0.4 percent (Cuong 2017; Vuong et al. 2011). Additionally, mental disorders due to substance addictions are increasing, and the average age of drug users is decreasing (Nguyen and Scannapieco 2008). However, as in many LMICs, Viet Nam has limited mental health resources, and the treatment gap is as high as 90 percent (Andrade et al. 2014; Collins and Saxena 2016; Minas and Lewis 2017; Niemi et al. 2010; Saxena 2016).

Around 12 percent of Vietnamese children and adolescents have a mental disorder. However, the reported prevalence varies from 8 to 29 percent, depending on the surveyed population (ODI and UNICEF Viet Nam 2018; Weiss et al. 2014). This translates to at least 3 million children and adolescents with mental health problems of sufficient severity to warrant treatment (ODI and UNICEF Viet Nam 2018; Weiss et al. 2014). Although the standard of living of most Vietnamese children and families has increased, the rapidly growing economy and globalization have also had negative consequences. Among others, these include significant issues within the family, such as decreases in parents' care and attention to their children, increases in parent-child conflicts, and drug and alcohol abuse, leading to increased risk of Vietnamese children developing mental health problems (UN Viet Nam Youth Theme Group 2010). Anxiety, depression, and attention-deficit/hyperactivity disorder (ADHD)[1] are the most common mental disorders among Vietnamese children and adolescents (ODI and UNICEF Viet Nam 2018). Mental health problems are the single most significant risk factor for functional impairment, and behavioral and mental health problems are associated with a 250 percent increase in impairment of school performance (Dang, Weiss, and Trung 2016). Approximately 0.75 percent of Vietnamese children have autism spectrum disorders (ASDs) (Hoang et al. 2019).[2] Among the population younger than 18 years, 2.2 percent have various levels of psychosocial disabilities (Viet Nam GSO 2016), pointing to the need to strengthen mental health care services that are tailored to children and adolescents in Viet Nam.

Among the elderly population, the number of people living with neurocognitive disorders, such as dementia and mental health problems, is increasing. Viet Nam is one of the fastest aging countries in the world, and this affects many aspects of society, including health and well-being (World Bank 2021b). It has been estimated that at least 20 percent of seniors suffer from a mental or neurological disease, accounting for 17.4 percent of the total years lived with disability (WHO 2017a). At the same time, multiple mental health burdens are documented among the older population in Viet Nam. Depression accounts for the highest percentage, an estimated 17 percent (Viet Nam MOH 2018). Additionally, dementia, stroke, and other disorders adversely affect older individuals' cognition and hamper their independence and functioning, making them vulnerable to abuse (Fang and Yan 2018), loneliness (Moyle et al. 2011), and depression (Snowden et al. 2015). Approximately 48 percent of older people have difficulties with memory, and almost 70 percent reported declining memory functioning over the past 12 months (World Bank 2021b). Dementia was estimated to affect more than 500,000 people in 2019, and it is projected that it will affect at least 1.5 million people in 2050 (Nichols et al. 2022). Additionally, about one in three older individuals has symptoms of chronic pain, and one in four suffers from sleep disturbances (Vu et al. 2020). Although the number of seniors with a mental or neurological disorder is increasing, their access to mental health care is limited. Two-thirds of the elderly population live in rural areas, and a majority of them are female (Pham et al. 2018). Yet, there is a lower availability of resources and relevant services in rural areas (Viet Nam MOH 2018), further demonstrating the need to develop the capacity of mental health care and human resources.

Women are at greater risk of mental health disorders, particularly in LMICs (Collier 2020; Freeman and Freeman 2013; Steel et al. 2014; United Nations 2015). In Viet Nam, there are significant mental health disparities between the genders, with women showing higher levels of all mental health–related problems, except alcohol dependency (Collier 2020). Among Vietnamese women attending general health clinics, 33 percent were found to have postpartum depressive symptoms, and 19 percent explicitly acknowledged having suicidal intentions (Fisher et al. 2004). These mental health problems negatively affect infants' physical health, their growth, the mother-infant relationship, and children's psychological development (Bennett et al. 2016; Madigan et al. 2018; Patel et al. 2004). Additionally, the prevalence of intimate partner violence during pregnancy ranges from 5.9 to 32.5 percent, depending on its form, and further worsens maternal mental disorders and adverse birth outcomes (Do et al. 2019).

The COVID-19 pandemic exacerbated the mental health crisis. The pandemic caused an increase in mental disorders and disrupted critical mental health services globally (WHO 2020a), and Viet Nam was not an exception. The pandemic made it clear that mental and physical health are not separate. By 2022, Viet Nam reported more than 10,500,000 confirmed cases of COVID-19 and more than 40,000 deaths due to the disease (WHO 2022). The pandemic affected the mental health of patients, health care workers, and the general population. Although many individuals who were infected with COVID-19 have recovered, others have experienced mental health problems as a direct consequence of the infection through long COVID with neuropsychiatric symptoms, or indirectly through the increased stress and instability the pandemic caused (Penninx et al. 2022). Among COVID-19 patients who were hospitalized, the rates of prevalence of depression and anxiety were 45 and 47 percent, respectively (Deng et al. 2021). Notably, 66.7 percent of COVID-19 patients who received oxygen therapy had symptoms of depression or anxiety, often related to long COVID (Viet Nam MOH 2021). Among health care workers in the COVID-19 hot spots, the prevalence of anxiety, depression, insomnia, and overall psychological problems were 26.84, 34.70, 34.53, and 46.48 percent, respectively (Tuan et al. 2021). Similarly, among the general population, it is estimated that the prevalence of major depressive disorder and anxiety disorders increased by 27 and 25 percent, respectively (Santomauro et al. 2021). The pandemic further increased the treatment gap for mental illnesses in Viet Nam. Indeed, while the need for mental health increased, the availability of mental health services was disrupted due to stringent restrictions or lockdowns (WHO 2020a).

## PROGRESS TOWARD ACHIEVING UNIVERSAL HEALTH COVERAGE FOR MENTAL DISORDERS

Viet Nam has made significant progress toward achieving universal health coverage (UHC), with an expanded health care network and increased public health spending. The health service delivery network has grown through a mixture of public and private resources. The country has more than 11,000 commune health stations, which form the grassroots of the public health care system in rural Viet Nam; regional public clinics; and nearly 32,000 private clinics at the primary care level. At the secondary and tertiary care levels, there are 1,451 hospitals, including about 300 private hospitals (Le, Govindaraj, and Bredenkamp 2020). Health insurance coverage increased from 13.4 percent of the population in 2000 to 90.9 percent in 2020. Although financial hardship has been mitigated, out-of-pocket payments at the point of care have remained high, at 44.9 percent of the costs in 2018. Catastrophic health expenditure has declined, and impoverishment due to health spending is low (Wagstaff, Flores, Hsu, et al. 2018; Wagstaff, Flores, Smitz, et al. 2018). Measured by the UHC service coverage index,[3] Viet Nam meets 73 percent of the population's health needs for essential health services, which is higher than Southeast Asia's average of 59 percent and the global average of 64 percent (WHO 2017b; WHO and World Bank 2017).

Due to better access to essential health services, the population's health outcomes have improved remarkably over the past three decades. The under-five mortality rate fell from 51 to 20.8 per 1,000 live births, and the maternal mortality ratio declined from 139 to 43 per 100,000 live births between 1990 and 2017 (World Bank 2020). Life expectancy at birth was 73.5 years in 2018, representing an increase of 5.5 years since 1999 (Viet Nam MOH 2019).

Although most Vietnamese have received benefits from UHC, people with mental illnesses still have limited access to quality mental health care services. Institutional approaches continue to dominate the mental health system, with psychiatric hospitals remaining the primary setting for the treatment and organization of mental health care (Minas and Lewis 2017). The most significant barriers to access to mental health care in rural areas are the limited availability of health professionals and access to treatment services (Van et al. 2021). In Viet Nam, people with serious mental illnesses[4] experience a prolonged delay in receiving a diagnosis of 11.5 months on average, negatively affecting treatment outcomes and resulting in a lower likelihood of long-term recovery (Nguyen et al. 2019). Although national health programs have been implemented at the grassroots level, treatment services are limited to people with severe psychiatric and neurological disorders, including schizophrenia, chronic epilepsy, and drug addiction. The remaining burden of common mental disorders, which affect about 15 percent of the population at any given time, has not yet been addressed. Out-of-pocket payments remain a significant issue for those with uncovered conditions (Nguyen et al. 2019; Niemi et al. 2010).

Although the social welfare network has been expanded, people with mental disorders still have limited access to social support. More than 324,000 people with severe mental disorders rely on monthly social assistance for support (Viet Nam MOLISA 2021). For those with severe and persistent mental illnesses, the national and provincial social affairs authorities have provided minimal support to residential centers (Minas and Lewis 2017). Together with psychiatric hospitals, welfare centers in the social sector contribute to improved coverage of psychiatric beds throughout the country. However, only a small percentage of people with mental disorders are admitted to these facilities in the health and social sectors (RTCCD 2014).

The social sector is moving from institutional support to community-based assistance. Due to the lack of adequate support for rehabilitation, many people with serious mental illnesses remain institutionalized for life because they are unable to recover, homeless, or jobless (Drake and Whitley 2014). Recognizing the limitations of the institutional approach, the national network of social protection and social work centers has gradually expanded its activities beyond institutional care to community-based services, including consultations, psycho-educational therapies, and other social activities. However, because it covers limited services, the social support network reaches only 30 percent of the targeted population (Viet Nam MOLISA 2018).

Due to stigmatization and discrimination, individuals who exhibit mental disorders and their family members seek care and support from informal systems rather than formal ones. In Viet Nam, people with mental illnesses and their families frequently experience public stigmatization and discrimination due to cultural factors (Ngo et al. 2014; Ta et al. 2016), posing an enormous challenge for the country's mental health care system. While patients and their families may be reluctant to disclose mental health problems, stigmatization of and discrimination against people with mental illnesses may also have a negative influence on help-seeking behavior, treatment outcomes, and rehabilitation of the affected individuals (Dockery et al. 2015; Martensen et al. 2020; Van der Ham et al. 2011). Low mental health literacy makes it difficult for laypeople to find effective mental health services (Dang et al. 2020). Therefore, people with mental disorders and their family members often seek treatment through the informal system (Ngo et al. 2014), including self-treatment; traditional medicines using herbs, acupuncture, massage, and various forms of exercise to promote the flow of inner energy; meditation; special diets; and religious or spiritual healing (Nguyen et al. 2018; Tuan et al. 2021). Stigmatization affects not only those with mental disorders and their relatives, but also psychiatric hospitals, as well as mental health care staff and psychiatrists (Angermeyer et al. 2017; Gaebel et al. 2015; Mungee et al. 2016), with men and religious individuals reporting more negative attitudes toward psychiatrists in Viet Nam (Ta et al. 2018).

There are unmet needs for community-based, integrated mental health care and support. Educational, employment, housing, and other social services for people with mental disorders are rarely available in communities, and the provision of support traditionally falls on families. Despite the increasing attention to integrated care, general questions still need to be answered about the multisectoral commitment to expand these services and integrate them into communities. Further highlighting the need to integrate social services and mental health needs, Viet Nam ranks low in the Asia-Pacific region on various indicators, including the environment, opportunities, and access to treatment and governance, as measured by the Mental Health Integration Index[5] (EIU 2016).

## NEED FOR A STUDY ON HUMAN RESOURCES FOR MENTAL HEALTH

There have been frequent calls to give mental health a higher profile on the global health and development agenda. Mental health care is often given the lowest priority (Alem 2002), and it receives less than 2 percent of national health budgets (WHO 2011). The United Nations General Assembly has adopted the 2030 Agenda for Sustainable Development, which promotes mental health and well-being. The Sustainable Development Goals (SDGs) recognize the importance of promoting mental health and well-being (SDG 3), as well as protecting the rights of people with mental health conditions and psychosocial disabilities

(SDGs 4, 8, 10, 11, and 17). The World Health Organization adopted the Comprehensive Mental Health Action Plan 2013–2030, a special initiative on UHC for mental health, in 2019–23, and the Thirteenth General Program of Work, 2019–23, with the Triple Billion targets, including mental health and well-being indicators (Saxena, Funk, and Chisholm 2015; WHO 2019a, 2019b). The World Bank engages countries and relevant stakeholders in urgent investment in mental health toward achieving UHC (World Bank 2018, 2021a). During the COVID-19 pandemic, international organizations repeated calls for further actions on mental health, including research as part of policy advocacy efforts (Holmes et al. 2020).

Viet Nam's national strategies and policies reflect an increasing awareness of mental health challenges and an emphasis on integrated care at the grassroots level for people with mental disorders. The Ruling Communist Party's resolution on enhancing health protection, care, and promotion calls for actions to improve Vietnamese people's health in terms of physical and mental conditions and well-being.[6] The National Masterplan for building and developing the grassroots health care network includes institutional and financial reforms to ensure that all the commune health stations can manage chronic conditions and monitor the health status of the entire population by 2030.[7] The Viet Nam Health Program proposes multisectoral actions to reduce substance abuse and develop a social rehabilitation service delivery network for those who need social protection, including individuals with disabilities due to mental health disorders.[8] The government has approved the program for community-based social assistance and rehabilitation to promote better health, social, educational, and legal support for people with mental disorders and children with autism.[9] Recently, the National Assembly updated the Laws on Medical Examination and Treatment, which enable the government to finance the development of the psychiatric workforce.

Although mental health research has grown significantly, there remains limited research evidence to inform mental health policy. On the demand side, studies provide a greater understanding of mental disorders among population groups and risk factors. On the supply side, considerable knowledge gaps in all the system building blocks remain a significant hindrance to strengthening the mental health care system. Notably, the lack of information on the mental health workforce makes it impossible to develop a feasible action plan for achieving universal mental health coverage. The need for an in-depth study on the mental health workforce toward achieving UHC has become more urgent as the COVID-19 pandemic has increased the burden of mental illnesses in Viet Nam and as the Ministry of Health is developing a National Action Plan to strengthen the mental health system.

## STUDY OBJECTIVES, FRAMEWORK, SCOPE, AND DATA COLLECTION METHODS

### Objectives

The study set out to achieve the following objectives:

- Understand the coverage of mental health service delivery.
- Assess the current status of the mental health workforce.

- Describe constraints in mental health education and training.
- Propose strategic priorities for transforming the workforce toward achieving UHC for mental health in Viet Nam.

## Framework

This descriptive study is underpinned by a conceptual framework that illustrates the interdependence of the following key elements: population needs, mental health service provision, mental health workforce, and mental health education and training (figure 1.1). The study examines the status of the mental health workforce and analyzes its constraints from both the supply side (training institutions) and the demand side (service providers) to formulate strategic priorities for achieving UHC for people with mental disorders.

## Scope

Aligned with the objectives, the study is comprised of four main parts:

(a) *Mental health service coverage in Viet Nam.* Chapter 2 reviews the organization and significant achievements of the mental health service delivery network at all levels in Viet Nam. Critical gaps and problems in service delivery for mental health are highlighted in terms of availability, accessibility, acceptability, and quality of service.

FIGURE 1.1

**Framework for assessing human resources for mental health service delivery toward achieving UHC in Viet Nam**

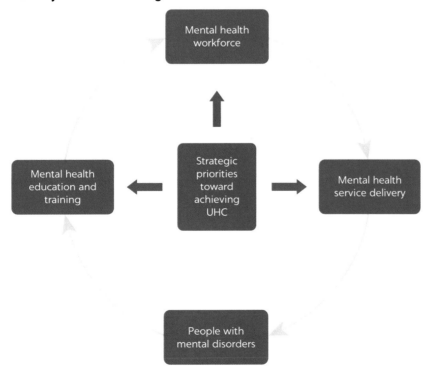

*Source:* Original figure for this report.
*Note:* UHC = universal health coverage.

(b) *Mental health workforce in Viet Nam.* Chapter 3 describes the current situation of the mental health workforce in Viet Nam. It analyzes critical issues, including shortages of various types of mental health professionals and their numbers (psychiatrists, psychologists, nurses, psychotherapists, social workers, occupational therapists, peer groups, and self-help groups, among others); maldistribution between levels of mental health care and regions (the urban and rural divide); and competency mismatch, job dissatisfaction, recruitment, and retention issues.

(c) *Mental health education and training in Viet Nam.* Chapter 4 describes the country's education and training system and identifies and analyzes constraints to future mental health workforce development from the supply side.

(d) *Conclusion and recommendations.* Chapter 5 proposes key strategic priorities and actions to be taken by government agencies and relevant stakeholders to strengthen the service delivery and workforce toward achieving UHC for mental health, based on the findings of this study.

## Data collection methods

The study combines rich qualitative and quantitative information from primary sources (online surveys, focus group discussions, and workshops) and secondary sources (literature review). Additionally, information was sourced from the websites of mental health service providers and mental health training institutions in Viet Nam and other countries. The data collection methods used in the study are summarized in table 1.1 and include the following:

- The literature review examined published and grey international literature (such as studies, reports, and guidelines) and published and grey literature from Viet Nam.
- Three online surveys were conducted between April and June 2021. The first collected data on human resources from 81 mental health facilities. The second collected information on professional status and job satisfaction from 1,121 mental health professionals in 10 cities and provinces. The third collected data on mental health education and training from 27 medical universities.
- Six group discussions with representatives of 10 provincial psychiatric hospitals were organized in June 2021. The discussions solicited information from

TABLE 1.1 **Data collection methods used for the study**

| | METHOD | | | |
| STUDY PART | LITERATURE REVIEW | ONLINE SURVEYS | FOCUS GROUP DISCUSSIONS | WORKSHOP |
| --- | --- | --- | --- | --- |
| Mental health service delivery (chapter 2) | + | | | |
| Mental health workforce (chapter 3) | + | + | + | |
| Mental health education and training (chapter 4) | + | + | + | + |
| Proposed strategic priorities (chapter 5) | + | | + | + |

*Source:* Original table for this report.

relevant stakeholders on constraints to future mental health workforce development and strategic priorities for transitioning the workforce toward achieving UHC for mental health.
- A workshop with representatives of mental health education institutions and mental health care facilities was organized in March 2023 to inform relevant stakeholders about the constraints to and recommendations for mental health workforce development from the supply and utilization sides.

## NOTES

1. ADHD is a neurodevelopmental disorder of childhood. Children with ADHD may have trouble with paying attention, controlling impulsive behaviors, or being overly active (https://www.cdc.gov/ncbddd/adhd/facts.html).
2. ASD is a developmental disorder caused by differences in the brain. People with ASD often have problems with social communication and interaction and restricted or repetitive behaviors or interests (https://www.cdc.gov/ncbddd/autism/signs.html).
3. The UHC service coverage index is a single indicator constructed from subindexes representing the four categories of reproductive, maternal, neonatal, and child health services; infectious diseases; noncommunicable diseases; and service capacity and access.
4. "Serious mental illness" is defined as one or more mental, behavioral, or emotional disorder(s) resulting in serious functional impairment, which substantially interferes with or limits one or more major life activities. Serious mental illness includes major depression, schizophrenia, bipolar disorder, obsessive-compulsive disorder, panic disorder, post-traumatic stress disorder, and borderline personality disorder (https://www.va.gov/PREVENTS/docs /PRE013_FactSheets_SeriousMentalillness_508.pdf).
5. The Mental Health Integration Index includes a set of 18 indicators grouped into the following four categories: (a) the environment for those with mental illness to be able to lead a full life; (b) access to medical help and services for people with mental illness; (c) the opportunities available to those with mental illness; and (d) governance of the system, including human rights issues and efforts to combat stigma.
6. Resolution No. 20/NQ-TW on enhancing health protection, care, and promotion in the new situation was issued by the Viet Nam Communist Party's Central Executive Committee on October 25, 2017.
7. The prime minister approved the National Masterplan for building and developing the grassroots health care network in the new situation under Decision 2348/QĐ-TTg on December 5, 2016.
8. The prime minister approved the Viet Nam Health Program by Decision 1092/QĐ-TTg on September 2, 2018.
9. The program on community-based social assistance and rehabilitation for people with mental disorders and children with autism was approved by the prime minister by Decision 1929/QĐ-TTg on November 25, 2021.

## REFERENCES

Alem, A. 2002. "Community-Based vs. Hospital-Based Mental Health Care: The Case of Africa." *World Psychiatry* 1 (2): 98–99. https://pubmed.ncbi.nlm.nih.gov/16946864.

Andrade, L. H., J. Alonso, Z. Mneimneh, J. E. Wells, A. Al-Hamzawi, G. Borges, E. Bromet, R. Bruffaerts, G. de Girolamo, R. de Graaf, S. Florescu, O. Gureje, H. R. Hinkov, C. Hu, Y. Huang, I. Hwang, R. Jin, E. G. Karam, V. Kovess-Masfety, . . . R. C. Kessler. 2014. "Barriers to Mental Health Treatment: Results from the WHO World Mental Health Surveys." *Psychological Medicine* 44 (6): 1303–17. https://doi.org/10.1017/S0033291713001943.

Angermeyer, M. C., S. Van Der Auwera, M. G. Carta, and G. Schomerus. 2017. "Public Attitudes towards Psychiatry and Psychiatric Treatment at the Beginning of the 21st Century: A Systematic Review and Meta-Analysis of Population Surveys." *World Psychiatry* 16 (1): 50–61.

Bennett, I. M., W. Schott, S. Krutikova, and J. R. Behrman. 2016. "Maternal Mental Health, and Child Growth and Development in Four Low-Income and Middle-Income Countries." *Journal of Epidemiology and Community Health* 70 (2): 168–73. https://doi.org/10.1136 /jech-2014-205311.

Bloom, D., E. Cafiero, E. Jané-Llopis, S. Abrahams-Gessel, L. Bloom, S. Fathima, A. Feigl, T. Gaziano, M. Mowafi, and A. Pandya. 2011. *The Global Economic Burden of Non-Communicable Diseases.* Geneva: World Economic Forum.

Charlson, F., M. van Ommeren, A. Flaxman, J. Cornett, H. Whiteford, and S. Saxena. 2019. "New WHO Prevalence Estimates of Mental Disorders in Conflict Settings: A Systematic Review and Meta-Analysis." *The Lancet* 394 (10194): 240–48.

Collier, K. M. 2020. "Explanatory Variables for Women's Increased Risk for Mental Health Problems in Vietnam." *Social Psychiatry and Psychiatric Epidemiology* 55 (3): 359.

Collins, P. Y., and S. Saxena. 2016. "Action on Mental Health Needs Global Cooperation." *Nature* 532 (7597): 25–27. https://doi.org/10.1038/532025a.

Cuong, T. V. 2017. "Mental Health Care in Vietnam." *American Journal of Psychiatry* 31: 287.

Dang, H. M., T. T. Lam, A. Dao, and B. Weiss. 2020. "Mental Health Literacy at the Public Health Level in Low and Middle Income Countries: An Exploratory Mixed Methods Study in Vietnam." *PLoS One* 15 (12): e0244573. https://doi.org/10.1371/journal.pone.0244573.

Dang, H.-M., B. Weiss, and L. T. Trung. 2016. "Functional Impairment and Mental Health Functioning among Vietnamese Children." *Social Psychiatry and Psychiatric Epidemiology* 51 (1): 39–47.

Deng, J., F. Zhou, W. Hou, Z. Silver, C. Y. Wong, O. Chang, E. Huang, and Q. K. Zuo. 2021. "The Prevalence of Depression, Anxiety, and Sleep Disturbances in COVID-19 Patients: A Meta-Analysis." *Annals of the New York Academy of Sciences* 1486 (1): 90–111. https://doi.org/10.1111 /nyas.14506.

Do, H. P., B. X. Tran, C. T. Nguyen, T. Van Vo, P. R. Baker, and M. P. Dunne. 2019. "Inter-Partner Violence during Pregnancy, Maternal Mental Health and Birth Outcomes in Vietnam: A Systematic Review." *Children and Youth Services Review* 96: 255–65.

Dockery, L., D. Jeffery, O. Schauman, P. Williams, S. Farrelly, O. Bonnington, J. Gabbidon, F. Lassman, G. Szmukler, G. Thornicroft, and S. Clement. 2015. "Stigma- and Non-Stigma-Related Treatment Barriers to Mental Healthcare Reported by Service Users and Caregivers." *Psychiatry Research* 228 (3): 612–19. https://doi.org/10.1016/j.psychres.2015.05.044.

Drake, R. E., and R. Whitley. 2014. "Recovery and Severe Mental Illness: Description and Analysis." *Canadian Journal of Psychiatry* 59 (5): 236–42. https://doi.org/10.1177/070674371 405900502.

EIU (Economist Intelligence Unit). 2016. *Mental Health and Integration: Provision for Supporting People with Mental Illness: A Comparison of 15 Asia-Pacific Countries.* London: EIU.

Fang, B., and E. Yan. 2018. "Abuse of Older Persons with Dementia: A Review of the Literature." *Trauma, Violence, & Abuse* 19 (2): 127–47. https://doi.org/10.1177/1524838016650185.

Fazel, S., and B. Runeson. 2020. "Suicide." *New England Journal of Medicine* 382 (3): 266–74. https://doi.org/10.1056/NEJMra1902944.

Fisher, J., M. Morrow, N. Nhu Ngoc, and L. Hoang Anh. 2004. "Prevalence, Nature, Severity and Correlates of Postpartum Depressive Symptoms in Vietnam." *BJOG: An International Journal of Obstetrics & Gynaecology* 111 (12): 1353–60.

Freeman, D., and J. Freeman. 2013. *The Stressed Sex: Uncovering the Truth about Men, Women, and Mental Health.* Oxford University Press.

Gaebel, W., H. Zäske, J. Zielasek, H.-R. Cleveland, K. Samjeske, H. Stuart, J. Arboleda-Florez, T. Akiyama, A. E. Baumann, O. Gureje, M. R. Jorge, M. Kastrup, Y. Suzuki, A. Tasman, T. M. Fidalgo, M. Jarema, S. B. Johnson, L. Kola, D. Krupchanka, . . . N. Sartorius. 2015. "Stigmatization of Psychiatrists and General Practitioners: Results of an International Survey." *European Archives of Psychiatry and Clinical Neuroscience* 265 (3): 189–97. https:// doi.org/10.1007/s00406-014-0530-8.

Hoang, V. M., T. V. Le, T. T. Q. Chu, B. N. Le, M. D. Duong, N. M. Thanh, V. Tac Pham, H. Minas, and T. T. H. Bui. 2019. "Prevalence of Autism Spectrum Disorders and Their Relation to Selected Socio-Demographic Factors among Children Aged 18-30 Months in Northern

Vietnam, 2017." *International Journal of Mental Health Systems* 13: article 29. https://doi .org/10.1186/s13033-019-0285-8.

Holmes, E. A., R. C. O'Connor, V. H. Perry, I. Tracey, S. Wessely, L. Arseneault, C. Ballard, H. Christensen, R. Cohen Silver, I. Everall, T. Ford, A. John, T. Kabir, K. King, I. Madan, S. Michie, A. K. Przybylski, R. Shafran, A. Sweeney, . . . E. Bullmore. 2020. "Multidisciplinary Research Priorities for the COVID-19 Pandemic: A Call for Action for Mental Health Science." *Lancet Psychiatry* 7 (6): 547–60. https://doi.org/10.1016/s2215-0366(20)30168-1.

*Lancet Global Health.* 2020. "Mental Health Matters." *The Lancet Global Health* 8 (11): e1352. https://doi.org/10.1016/S2214-109X(20)30432-0.

Le, S. M., R. Govindaraj, and C. Bredenkamp. 2020. *Public-Private Partnerships for Health in Vietnam: Issues and Options.* International Development in Focus. Washington, DC: World Bank. https://doi.org/10.1596/978-1-4648-1574-4.

Madigan, S., H. Oatley, N. Racine, R. M. P. Fearon, L. Schumacher, E. Akbari, J. E. Cooke, and G. M. Tarabulsy. 2018. "A Meta-Analysis of Maternal Prenatal Depression and Anxiety on Child Socioemotional Development." *Journal of the American Academy of Child and Adolescent Psychiatry* 57 (9): 645–57. e648. https://doi.org/10.1016/j.jaac.2018.06.012.

Martensen, L. K., E. Hahn, C. T. Duc, G. Schomerus, K. Böge, M. Dettling, M. C. Angermeyer, and T. M. T. Ta. 2020. "Impact and Differences of Illness Course Perception on the Desire for Social Distance towards People with Symptoms of Depression or Schizophrenia in Hanoi, Vietnam." *Asian Journal of Psychiatry* 50: 101973.

Minas, H., and M. Lewis. 2017. *Mental Health in Asia and the Pacific: Historical and Cultural Perspectives.* New York: Springer.

Moyle, W., U. Kellett, A. Ballantyne, and N. Gracia. 2011. "Dementia and Loneliness: An Australian Perspective." *Journal of Clinical Nursing* 20 (9-10): 1445–53. https://doi .org/10.1111/j.1365-2702.2010.03549.x.

Mungee, A., A. Zieger, G. Schomerus, T. M. T. Ta, M. Dettling, M. C. Angermeyer, and E. Hahn. 2016. "Attitude towards Psychiatrists: A Comparison between Two Metropolitan Cities in India." *Asian Journal of Psychiatry* 22: 140–44.

Ngo, V. K., B. Weiss, T. Lam, T. Dang, T. Nguyen, and M. H. Nguyen. 2014. "The Vietnam Multicomponent Collaborative Care for Depression Program: Development of Depression Care for Low- and Middle-Income Nations." *Journal of Cognitive Psychotherapy* 28 (3): 156–67.

Nguyen, H. V., H. T. H. Do, V. T. A. Le, and N.-A. Mai. 2018. "Reviewing the Latest National Policies and Services for People with Severe Mental Health Disorders in Government-Funded Institutions in Vietnam and Policy Recommendations for Service Improvements." *Asia Pacific Journal of Social Work and Development* 28 (1): 56–68.

Nguyen, V. T., and M. Scannapieco. 2008. "Drug Abuse in Vietnam: A Critical Review of the Literature and Implications for Future Research." *Addiction* 103 (4): 535–43.

Nguyen, T., T. Tran, S. Green, A. Hsueh, T. Tran, H. Tran, and J. Fisher. 2019. "Delays to Diagnosis among People with Severe Mental Illness in Rural Vietnam, a Population-Based Cross-Sectional Survey." *BMC Psychiatry* 19: 385. https://doi.org/10.1186/s12888-019-2367-1.

Nichols, E., J. D. Steinmetz, S. E. Vollset, K. Fukutaki, J. Chalek, F. Abd-Allah, A. Abdoli, A. Abualhasan, E. Abu-Gharbieh, T. T. Akram, H. Al Hamad, F. Alahdab, F. M. Alanezi, V. Alipour, S. Almustanyir, H. Amu, I. Ansari, J. Arabloo, T. Ashraf, . . . T. Vos. 2022. "Estimation of the Global Prevalence of Dementia in 2019 and Forecasted Prevalence in 2050: An Analysis for the Global Burden of Disease Study 2019." *The Lancet Public Health* 7 (2): e105–e125. https://doi.org/10.1016/S2468-2667(21)00249-8.

Niemi, M., H. T. Thanh, T. Tuan, and T. Falkenberg. 2010. "Mental Health Priorities in Vietnam: A Mixed-Methods Analysis." *BMC Health Services Research* 10 (1): 1–10.

ODI and UNICEF Viet Nam (Overseas Development Institute and United Nations Children's Fund Viet Nam). 2018. *Mental Health and Psychosocial Wellbeing of Children and Young People in Selected Provinces and Cities in Viet Nam.* Hanoi: UNICEF Viet Nam.

Otte, C., S. M. Gold, B. W. Penninx, C. M. Pariante, A. Etkin, M. Fava, D. C. Mohr, and A. F. Schatzberg. 2016. "Major Depressive Disorder." *Nature Reviews Disease Primers* 2 (1): 1–20.

Patel, V., D. Chisholm, R. Parikh, F. J. Charlson, L. Degenhardt, T. Dua, A. J. Ferrari, S. Hyman, R. Laxminarayan, C. Levin, C. Lund, M. E. Medina Mora, I. Petersen, J. Scott, R. Shidhaye, L. Vijayakumar, G. Thornicroft, and H. Whiteford. 2016. "Addressing the Burden of Mental, Neurological, and Substance Use Disorders: Key Messages from Disease Control Priorities, 3rd Edition." *The Lancet* 387 (10028): 1672–85. https://doi.org/10.1016/S0140-6736 (15)00390-6.

Patel, V., A. Rahman, K. S. Jacob, and M. Hughes. 2004. "Effect of Maternal Mental Health on Infant Growth in Low-Income Countries: New Evidence from South Asia." *BMJ* 328 (7443): 820–23. https://doi.org/10.1136/bmj.328.7443.820.

Penninx, B. W., M. E. Benros, R. S. Klein, and C. H. Vinker. 2022. "How COVID-19 Shaped Mental Health: From Infection to Pandemic Effects." *Nature Medicine* 28 (10): 2027–37. https://doi.org/10.1038/s41591-022-02028-2.

Pham, T., N. T. T. Nguyen, S. B. ChieuTo, T. L. Pham, T. X. Nguyen, H. T. T. Nguyen, T. N. Nguyen, T. H. T. Nguyen, Q. N. Nguyen, B. X. Tran, L. H. Nguyen, G. H. Ha, C. A. Latkin, C. S. H. Ho, R. C. M. Ho, A. T. Nguyen, and H. T. T. Vu. 2018. "Sex Differences in Quality of Life and Health Services Utilization among Elderly People in Rural Vietnam." *International Journal of Environmental Research and Public Health* 16 (1). https://doi.org/10.3390/ijerph16010069.

Richardson, L. K., A. B. Amstadter, D. G. Kilpatrick, M. T. Gaboury, T. L. Tran, L. T. Trung, N. T. Tam, T. Tuan, L. T. Buoi, and T. T. Ha. 2010. "Estimating Mental Distress in Vietnam: The Use of the SRQ-20." *International Journal of Social Psychiatry* 56 (2): 133–42.

RTCCD (Research and Training Centre for Community Development). 2014. *Baseline Survey on Mental Healthcare System for People with Mental Illness in Thanh Hoa and Ben Tre Provinces.* Hanoi: RTCCD.

Santomauro, D. F., A. M. Mantilla Herrera, J. Shadid, P. Zheng, C. Ashbaugh, D. M. Pigott, C. Abbafati, C. Adolph, J. O. Amlag, A. Y. Aravkin, B. L. Bang-Jensen, G. J. Bertolacci, S. S. Bloom, R. Castellano, E. Castro, S. Chakrabarti, J. Chattopadhyay, R. M. Cogen, J. K. Collins, . . . A. J. Ferrari. 2021. "Global Prevalence and Burden of Depressive and Anxiety Disorders in 204 Countries and Territories in 2020 Due to the COVID-19 Pandemic." *The Lancet* 398 (10312): 1700–12. https://doi.org/10.1016/S0140-6736(21)02143-7.

Saxena, S. 2016. *mhGAP Intervention Guide for Mental, Neurological and Substance Use Disorders in Non-Specialized Health Settings Version 2.0.* Geneva: World Health Organization.

Saxena, S., M. Funk, and D. Chisholm. 2015. "Comprehensive Mental Health Action Plan 2013–2020." *Eastern Mediterranean Health Journal* 21 (7): 461–63.

Scott, K. M., C. Lim, A. Al-Hamzawi, J. Alonso, R. Bruffaerts, J. M. Caldas-de-Almeida, S. Florescu, G. De Girolamo, C. Hu, and P. De Jonge. 2016. "Association of Mental Disorders with Subsequent Chronic Physical Conditions: World Mental Health Surveys from 17 Countries." *JAMA Psychiatry* 73 (2): 150–58.

Snowden, M. B., D. C. Atkins, L. E. Steinman, J. F. Bell, L. L. Bryant, C. Copeland, and A. L. Fitzpatrick. 2015. "Longitudinal Association of Dementia and Depression." *American Journal of Geriatric Psychiatry* 23 (9): 897–905. https://doi.org/10.1016/j.jagp.2014.09.002.

Steel, Z., C. Marnane, C. Iranpour, T. Chey, J. W. Jackson, V. Patel, and D. Silove. 2014. "The Global Prevalence of Common Mental Disorders: A Systematic Review and Meta-Analysis 1980-2013." *International Journal of Epidemiology* 43 (2): 476–93. https://doi.org/10.1093/ije/dyu038.

Ta, T. M. T., K. Böge, T. D. Cao, G. Schomerus, T. D. Nguyen, M. Dettling, A. Mungee, L. K. Martensen, A. Diefenbacher, M. C. Angermeyer, and E. Hahn. 2018. "Public Attitudes towards Psychiatrists in the Metropolitan Area of Hanoi, Vietnam." *Asian Journal of Psychiatry* 32: 44–49. https://doi.org/10.1016/j.ajp.2017.11.031.

Ta, T. M. T., A. Zieger, G. Schomerus, T. D. Cao, M. Dettling, X. T. Do, A. Mungee, A. Diefenbacher, M. C. Angermeyer, and E. Hahn. 2016. "Influence of Urbanity on Perception of Mental Illness Stigma: A Population Based Study in Urban and Rural Hanoi, Vietnam." *International Journal of Social Psychiatry* 62 (8): 685–95.

Tuan, N. Q., N. D. Phuong, D. X. Co, D. N. Son, L. Q. Chinh, N. H. Dung, P. T. Thach, N. Q. Thai, T. A. Thu, N. A. Tuan, B. V. San, V. S. Tung, N. V. An, D. N. Khanh, V. H. Long, N. Tai, T. Muoi, N. D. Vinh, N. T. Thien, . . . N. V. Tuan. 2021. "Prevalence and Factors Associated with Psychological Problems of Healthcare Workforce in Vietnam: Findings from COVID-19

Hotspots in the National Second Wave." *Healthcare* (Basel) 9 (6). https://doi.org/10.3390/healthcare9060718.

UNDP (United Nations Development Programme). 2022. *Human Development Report 2021/2022: Uncertain Times, Unsettled Lives: Shaping Our Future in a Transforming World.* New York: UNDP.

United Nations. 2015. *Sustainable Development Goals.* New York: United Nations. https://sdgs.un.org/goals.

UN Viet Nam Youth Theme Group. 2010. "United Nations Position Paper on Young People in Viet Nam 2008–2010." United Nations, New York.

Van, N. H. N., N. Thi Khanh Huyen, M. T. Hue, N. T. Luong, P. Quoc Thanh, D. M. Duc, V. Thi Thanh Mai, and T. T. Hong. 2021. "Perceived Barriers to Mental Health Services among the Elderly in the Rural of Vietnam: A Cross-Sectional Survey in 2019." *Health Services Insights* 14: 11786329211026035.

Van der Ham, L., P. Wright, T. V. Van, V. D. Doan, and J. E. Broerse. 2011. "Perceptions of Mental Health and Help-Seeking Behavior in an Urban Community in Vietnam: An Explorative Study." *Community Mental Health Journal* 47 (5): 574–82.

Viet Nam GSO (General Statistics Office of Viet Nam). 2016. *The National Survey on People with Disabilities 2016.* VDS2016 Final Report. Hanoi: Viet Nam GSO.

Viet Nam MOH (Ministry of Health of Viet Nam). 2018. *The Program Targeting Health–Population Program 2016–2020: New Features in Fund Management and Utilization.* Hanoi: Viet Nam MOH.

Viet Nam MOH (Ministry of Health of Viet Nam). 2019. *Health Statistics Yearbook 2017–2018.* Hanoi: Medical Publishing House.

Viet Nam MOH (Ministry of Health of Viet Nam). 2021. "Ho Chi Minh City: 20 Percent of COVID-19 Patients Suffered from Depression and 66.7 Percent of Patients Undertaking Ventilator Suffered from Anxiety Disorders." Viet Nam MOH, Hanoi. https://moh.gov.vn/hoat-dong-cua-dia-phuong/-/asset_publisher/gHbla8vOQDuS/content/tp-hcm-20-benh-nhan-covid-19-bi-tram-cam-66-7-benh-nhan-tung-tho-may-bi-roi-loan-lo-au.

Viet Nam MOLISA (Ministry of Labour, Invalids, and Social Affairs of Viet Nam). 2018. *Evaluation Report: The Implementation of the Legal Framework on Social Works.* Hanoi: Viet Nam MOLISA.

Viet Nam MOLISA (Ministry of Labour, Invalids, and Social Affairs of Viet Nam). 2021. *Draft Master Plan for the Social Welfare Network in the Period of 2021–2030 with a Vision to 2050.* Hanoi: Viet Nam MOLISA.

Vigo, D., G. Thornicroft, and R. Atun. 2016. "Estimating the True Global Burden of Mental Illness." *The Lancet Psychiatry* 3 (2): 171–78.

Vu, N. C., M. T. Tran, L. T. Dang, C.-L. Chei, and Y. Saito (eds.). 2020. *Aging and Health in Viet Nam.* Central Jakarta, Indonesia: Economic Research Institute for ASEAN and East Asia.

Vuong, D. A., E. Van Ginneken, J. Morris, S. T. Ha, and R. Busse. 2011. "Mental Health in Vietnam: Burden of Disease and Availability of Services." *Asian Journal of Psychiatry* 4 (1): 65–70.

Wagstaff, A., G. Flores, J. Hsu, M.-F. Smitz, K. Chepynoga, L. R. Buisman, K. van Wilgenburg, and P. Eozenou. 2018. "Progress on Catastrophic Health Spending in 133 Countries: A Retrospective Observational Study." *The Lancet Global Health* 6 (2): e169–e179.

Wagstaff, A., G. Flores, M.-F. Smitz, J. Hsu, K. Chepynoga, and P. Eozenou. 2018. "Progress on Impoverishing Health Spending in 122 Countries: A Retrospective Observational Study." *The Lancet Global Health* 6 (2): e180–e192. https://doi.org/10.1016/S2214-109X(17)30486-2.

Walker, E. R., R. E. McGee, and B. G. Druss. 2015. "Mortality in Mental Disorders and Global Disease Burden Implications: A Systematic Review and Meta-Analysis." *JAMA Psychiatry* 72 (4): 334–41. https://doi.org/10.1001/jamapsychiatry.2014.2502.

Weiss, B., M. Dang, L. Trung, M. C. Nguyen, N. T. H. Thuy, and A. Pollack. 2014. "A Nationally Representative Epidemiological and Risk Factor Assessment of Child Mental Health in Vietnam." *International Perspectives in Psychology* 3 (3): 139–53.

WHO (World Health Organization). 2011. *Mental Health Atlas 2011.* Geneva: WHO.

WHO (World Health Organization). 2017a. *Mental Health of Older Adults.* Geneva: WHO.

WHO (World Health Organization). 2017b. *Tracking Universal Health Coverage: 2017 Global Monitoring Report*. Geneva: WHO.

WHO (World Health Organization). 2019a. *The Thirteenth General Programme of Work 2019–2023*. Geneva: WHO. https://www.who.int/about/what-we-do/thirteenth-general-programme-of-work-2019---2023.

WHO (World Health Organization). 2019b. *The WHO Special Initiative for Mental Health (Vietnam Central Steering Committee for the 2019 Population and Housing Census): Universal Health Coverage for Mental Health*. Geneva: WHO.

WHO (World Health Organization). 2020a. "COVID-19 Disrupting Mental Health Services in Most Countries: WHO Survey." WHO, Geneva. https://www.who.int/news/item/05-10-2020-covid-19-disrupting-mental-health-services-in-most-countries-who-survey.

WHO (World Health Organization). 2020b. "World Mental Health Day: An Opportunity to Kick-Start a Massive Scale-up in Investment in Mental Health." WHO, Geneva (accessed April 20, 2022), https://www.who.int/news/item/27-08-2020-world-mental-health-day-an-opportunity-to-kick-start-a-massive-scale-up-in-investment-in-mental-health.

WHO (World Health Organization). 2022. "WHO (COVID-19) Homepage." WHO, Geneva (accessed April 22, 2022), https://covid19.who.int/region/wpro/country/vn.

WHO and World Bank (World Health Organization and World Bank). 2017. *Tracking Universal Health Coverage: 2017 Global Monitoring Report*. Washington, DC: World Health Organization and World Bank.

World Bank. 2018. *Moving the Needle: Mental Health Stories from around the World*. Washington, DC: World Bank.

World Bank. 2020. *World Development Indicators*. Washington, DC: World Bank.

World Bank. 2021a. *Universal Health Coverage*. Washington, DC: World Bank. https://www.worldbank.org/en/topic/universalhealthcoverage#1.

World Bank. 2021b. *Vietnam: Adapting to an Aging Society*. Washington, DC: World Bank.

# 2 Mental Health Service Coverage in Viet Nam

## INTRODUCTION

This chapter provides an overview of the mental health service delivery networks in Viet Nam across sectors, encompassing a review of each system's organization and significant achievements at the institutional and community levels. The chapter highlights critical gaps and problems in mental health service delivery in terms of availability, accessibility, and quality of service.

## OVERVIEW OF MENTAL HEALTH SERVICE DELIVERY NETWORKS

In Viet Nam, mental health services are delivered through four interconnected domains: health care, social welfare, education, and informal systems. The health system is structured into four levels of care: commune, district, provincial, and central. The social system includes six types of service providers—counseling hotlines, counseling centers, social work centers, social protection centers, mental health rehabilitation centers, and drug de-addiction centers—which offer institutional or community-based care. The education system aims to provide services for children and adolescents at schools. Individuals, families, and community members often act as informal caregivers (figure 2.1).

## MENTAL HEALTH CARE SERVICES IN THE HEALTH SECTOR

Mental health care services in the health sector include hospital-based services and community-based services through a public-private mix.

### Hospital-based mental health care services

Mental health care service delivery in Viet Nam is mainly undertaken in psychiatric hospitals. Increased investment in psychiatric hospitals over the past decades improved the availability of specialized psychiatric services in most of the country's 63 provinces. There are five psychiatric hospitals and institutes at

FIGURE 2.1

**Key mental health service providers across sectors in Viet Nam**

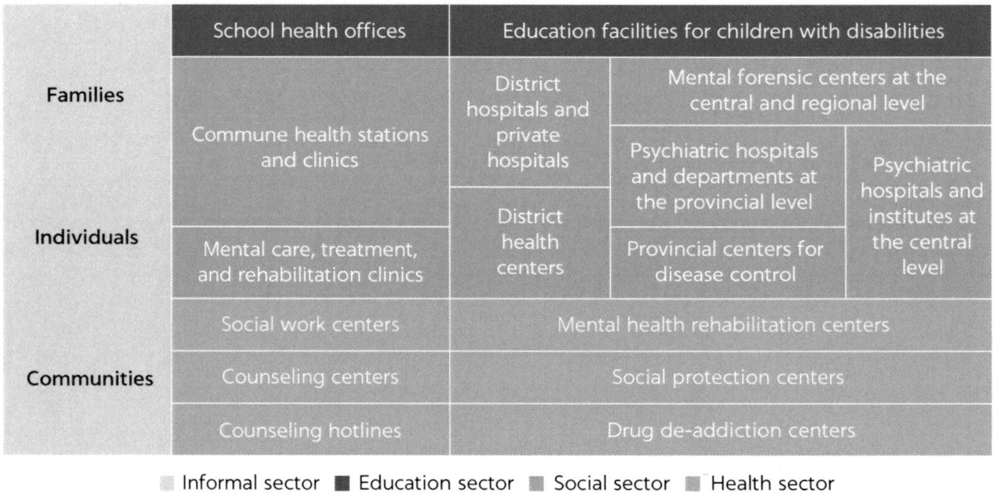

| | School health offices | Education facilities for children with disabilities | | |
|---|---|---|---|---|
| **Families** | Commune health stations and clinics | District hospitals and private hospitals | Mental forensic centers at the central and regional level | |
| | | | Psychiatric hospitals and departments at the provincial level | Psychiatric hospitals and institutes at the central level |
| **Individuals** | Mental care, treatment, and rehabilitation clinics | District health centers | Provincial centers for disease control | |
| **Communities** | Social work centers | Mental health rehabilitation centers | | |
| | Counseling centers | Social protection centers | | |
| | Counseling hotlines | Drug de-addiction centers | | |

▨ Informal sector  ■ Education sector  ▨ Social sector  ▨ Health sector

*Source:* Original figure for this report.

the central level and 43 psychiatric hospitals at the provincial level. The number of psychiatric hospital beds reached 10,000 in 2021, equivalent to 10.3 psychiatric hospital beds per 100,000 population. This number was a significant increase from 6.18 psychiatric hospital beds per 100,000 population in 2006 (WHO and Viet Nam MOH 2006), and it is close to the global average of 10.8 and far above the low- and middle-income country average of 3.8 (WHO 2021). Additionally, 28 general hospitals have a psychiatric department or ward, accounting for 0.19 bed for psychiatric patients per 100,000 population. Only 7 percent of the country's hospital beds for patients with mental illnesses are integrated into general hospitals, which is lower than the share in the Republic of Korea, at 14 percent (Go et al. 2020); China, at 21 percent (Xia et al. 2021); Japan, at 25 percent; the United States, at 54 percent (McCance-Katz 2018); and Germany, at 71 percent (WHO 2019).

The uneven availability of psychiatric hospital resources translates into unequal access to mental health services across the country's provinces and by socioeconomic status. While the top five cities and provinces have more than 20 psychiatric hospital beds per 100,000 population, five provinces have less than 1 bed per 100,000 population. The geographic variation in the number of psychiatric beds is substantial, as shown in map 2.1 and figure 2.2. The Central Highlands region has only 3.5 psychiatric hospital beds per 100,000 population, threefold lower than the national average. The Northern Upland region has 6.1 psychiatric hospital beds per 100,000 population, 2.7 times fewer than the nearby Red River Delta region. The limited availability of psychiatric hospitals is especially evident for the Vietnamese population in mountainous areas, reflecting the geographic barriers to accessing mental health care services.

Furthermore, there is an urban-rural divide, in which patients living in rural areas have less access to psychiatric hospital care. As psychiatric hospitals are often located in urban or suburban settings, the individuals residing in these areas have greater access to mental health care, including psychiatrists, medications, facilities, and psychosocial interventions (Humphries et al. 2015).

MAP 2.1

**Total psychiatric hospital and residential beds per 100,000 population in Viet Nam mainland, 2021**

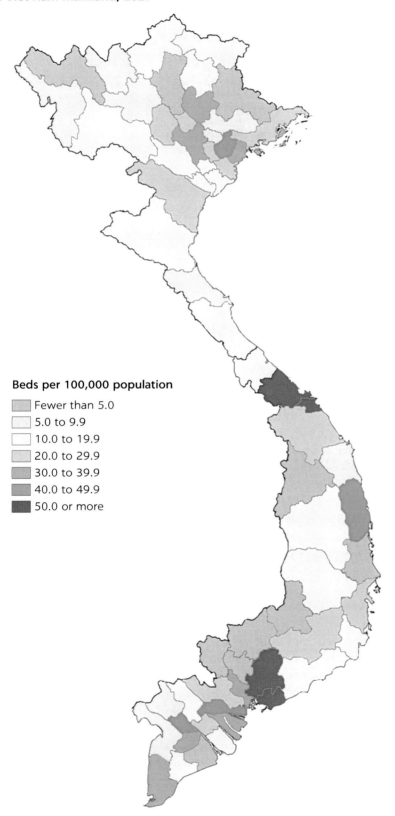

Beds per 100,000 population

- Fewer than 5.0
- 5.0 to 9.9
- 10.0 to 19.9
- 20.0 to 29.9
- 30.0 to 39.9
- 40.0 to 49.9
- 50.0 or more

*Source:* Original map for this report.

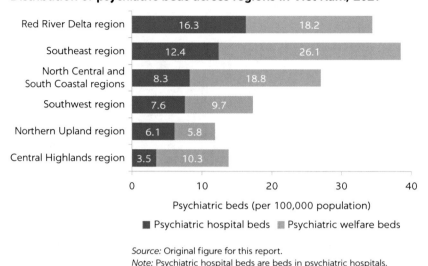

FIGURE 2.2

**Distribution of psychiatric beds across regions in Viet Nam, 2021**

Source: Original figure for this report.
Note: Psychiatric hospital beds are beds in psychiatric hospitals.
Psychiatric welfare beds are beds in psychiatric welfare centers.

The most significant barriers in rural areas are the limited availability and accessibility of health professionals and services (Van et al. 2021). Among patients visiting district-level health facilities, 52.5 percent experience distance-related distress (World Bank 2019). To seek better health care at central and provincial psychiatric hospitals, patients and their caregivers from rural communities must travel longer distances and pay more for expenses; therefore, they are less likely to seek help or continue treatment. The statistics show that there are urban-rural disparities in mental health outcomes, with higher rates of psychiatric disabilities among people living in rural areas (Viet Nam GSO 2016).

The quality of mental health care is another concern. The psychiatric hospitals in Viet Nam follow the "biomedical model" in general, focusing mainly on psychopharmacological treatment. The use of psychiatric medications, and especially the application of polypharmacy treatments, has increased over time. Although a combination of nonpharmacological interventions, such as psychotherapy and psychosocial rehabilitation, has been proved effective and endorsed, the supply of nonpharmacological interventions remains limited (Böge et al. 2018; Minas and Lewis 2017). The quality of services in Viet Nam is generally poor by international standards (Nguyen, Tran, Green, et al. 2019). The "biopsychosocial model"—using person-centered treatment approaches and shared decision-making—is supported by evidence from research studies (Babalola, Pia, and Ross 2017; Boardman and Dave 2020). However, treatment in psychiatric hospitals in Viet Nam faces systematic challenges, including skill mix imbalance and lack of financial incentives to deliver modern integrated care.

The overprovision of and increasing spending on psychiatric hospitals have triggered arguments about efficiency in mental health care. Over the past decades, provincial authorities have promoted highly specialized mental health care by establishing psychiatric hospitals rather than strengthening the psychiatric departments in general hospitals. Questions remain about how specialized psychiatric hospitals can coordinate patient care, as many mental disorders are comorbid or associated with other chronic medical illnesses.

Moreover, stigma toward mental disorders tends to be lower if treatment is integrated into general health care. While Viet Nam has been increasing the number of psychiatric hospital beds, high-income countries have been "deinstitutionalizing"—moving people out of psychiatric hospitals toward care in the community. In some countries, such as Italy, the United Kingdom, and the United States, the deinstitutionalization process started over 50 years ago (OECD 2014).

Another concern is related to the primary purpose of mental health care: helping people with serious mental illnesses (SMIs) to recover and live in their community. Throughout the country, only one psychiatric hospital implements the day care model, and 50 percent of provincial-level mental health facilities and 61 percent of district-level mental health facilities offer outpatient services for people with mental disorders to access treatment while staying with their families (Viet Nam MOH 2023). The remaining psychiatric hospitals treat the psychiatric symptoms of SMIs through inpatient services, with patients staying in the hospital until they are discharged with limited recovery support. Only 11 and 37 percent of psychiatric hospitals offer occupational therapy and work therapy, respectively (Viet Nam MOH 2023). Although they are managing critical resources for mental health care, psychiatric hospitals face challenges in expanding their services beyond the institutional borders to the communities in which people with SMIs struggle to integrate.

## Community mental health services

In addition to hospitals, the public health network has been expanded extensively at the grassroots level, and almost all the communes have a commune health station (CHS). Typically, each CHS is equipped with four or five beds and essential equipment and staffed with a general physician, an assistant physician, a nurse, a midwife, and an assistant pharmacist. In 2018, 94.5 percent of the CHSs had a midwife or pediatric-obstetric assistant physician, 90.8 percent of the CHSs had a physician serving full time or part time, and 81 percent of the communes met the national criteria for commune health (Viet Nam MOH 2019). However, these structural benchmarks do not ensure that CHSs can manage specific conditions, particularly noncommunicable diseases. Only 48.8 percent of CHSs can perform at least 80 percent of the professional techniques on the regulated service list (Viet Nam MOH 2020).

More than 11,100 CHSs deliver essential mental health services at the community level. In 2000, the Ministry of Health launched the community mental health program (CMHP), starting with a focus on schizophrenia, then expanding to chronic epilepsy, and recently depression. The CMHP consists of three levels of interactions: primary health centers connected to the districts, provincial psychiatric hospitals, and national psychiatric hospitals. The CMHP aims to support recognition of mental disorders, basic psychiatric treatment, and relapse prevention, thus reducing risk and disability (Ng et al. 2011b). Over the past 20 years, the CMHP has been implemented in all 63 provinces. It has built the capacities of health workers, particularly psychiatrists; enhanced community mental health practices; and improved access to diagnosis and treatment services for people with schizophrenia and chronic epilepsy, especially for those who live in remote areas (Cuong 2017). To date, the community health services under the CMHP have been embedded in primary health care activities and helped to accelerate progress toward integrating the informal workforce into the mental health care system. As an integral part of the health service package at the grassroots level,[1] the CMHP has also raised public awareness and understanding of mental illness (Ng et al. 2011a). Furthermore, the methadone maintenance therapy program has been implemented in 57 provinces as part of community-based treatment services (Khue et al. 2017).

However, the scope of the mental health services provided by CHSs is limited. CHSs mainly focus on providing and revising pharmacological treatment for patients with schizophrenia, chronic epilepsy, and depression, and providing methadone maintenance therapy. The CMHP requires an assigned CHS staff member to refer individuals with mental health issues to the primary health center for diagnosis, follow up patients discharged from hospitals, renew prescriptions, provide medications initially approved by the hospital, and report to the district health center every month. A similar approach has been piloted for treating depression in several provinces; however, due to the lack of financial and human resources, CHSs have not systematically integrated the treatment of depression (Tran, La, and Nguyen 2007). The commonly available medications at CHSs for people with mental illnesses include first- and second-generation antipsychotics (chlorpromazine, haloperidol, levomepromazine, clozapine, risperidone, and olanzapine), antidepressants (amitriptyline and sertraline), and methadone.

Beyond the provision of medications, most CHSs cannot deliver other mental health services, such as screening, psychotherapy, relapse prevention, rehabilitation, or recovery support. A recent assessment in six provinces revealed that only 42.6 percent of trained primary health care teams perform mental health screening services at CHSs (CEHS 2020). The CMHP made an effort to expand services to children with autism spectrum disorders (ASDs) and attention-deficit/hyperactivity disorder, but it faced a challenging shortage of staff and experience in dealing with pediatric mental disorders (Cuong 2017). A few districts have recently adopted collaborative stepped care, community-based interventions, including psychotherapy, psychoeducation, counseling, and yoga for depression management at the CHSs. Despite promising evidence of effectiveness from the pilot phase, the scalability and long-term sustainability of the collaborative stepped care model for depression management at the primary health care level remain uncertain due to structural factors (Do, Nguyen, and Tran 2022; Ngo et al. 2014; Nguyen, Tran, Green, et al. 2020; Niemi et al. 2016). Widespread concerns about human and financial resources for CHSs to deliver appropriate mental health services have been raised since the CMHP was integrated into the Viet Nam Health–Population Program in 2017,[2] which resulted in a drastic reduction of financing for other professional activities (Viet Nam MOH 2018).

CHSs mainly rely on the district health center's support (training, drugs, materials, and operational budget) to maintain mental health services. Each district has a district health center, and each district health center assigns staff to be in charge of the community mental health program. This organizational arrangement translates into about 700 health professionals delivering outpatient mental health services at the district level. They provide mental disorder diagnoses, refer patients with mental disorders to the provincial level, and follow up patient care and treatment at the commune level. In addition to clinical work, these health professionals take on program management responsibilities, including planning, training, monitoring, supervision, reporting, drug estimation, distribution, and so forth.

At the provincial level, the Centers for Disease Control (CDC) is usually the focal institution for managing various public health programs, including the CMHP. Almost all of the country's 63 cities and provinces have constituted a CDC by consolidating preventive health centers. However, less than half of the CDCs have established a mental health department that would enable them to expand their scope of work beyond management of the CMHP to provide mental health care services directly to patients at clinics and in the community. Although they focus on inpatient care, provincial psychiatric hospitals may offer community mental health services through outreach activities on an ad-hoc basis.

### Private sector participation in mental health care services

While public health institutions face constraints to delivering community mental health services, private clinics are slowly expanding. Numerous private mental health clinics operate in larger metropolitan cities, like Hanoi and Ho Chi Minh City. Part-time and retired psychiatrists, psychologists, and educators provide outpatient mental health care services to children with ASD and attention-deficit/hyperactivity disorder and people with mental disorders. However, no private psychiatric hospitals have been established for patients with SMIs. Since there is no government subsidy for these services, the private mental health clinics serve a small subpopulation in need, who can pay out of pocket.

## MENTAL HEALTH CARE AND REHABILITATION IN THE SOCIAL SECTOR

Mental health care and rehabilitation in the social sector includes institution-based services, community-based services, and the drug addiction treatment network.

### Institution-based care and rehabilitation for individuals with SMIs

In line with the health care system, the social protection network for people with mental disorders has largely followed the institutional approach. As they were built during wartime, the social welfare facilities initially targeted people with severe brain injuries, then gradually expanded their services to people with SMIs. In 2020, more than 100 social institutions, including 31 psychiatric rehabilitation centers and more than 70 general social protection centers (SPCs), provided care for 15,800 individuals with SMIs, covering nearly 5 percent of all people with SMIs requiring social support assistance (Viet Nam MOLISA 2021).

Psychiatric rehabilitation has been improved over the past decade, but service coverage is still insufficient. Thirty-one psychiatric care and rehabilitation centers were established in Viet Nam by 2020, which was a twofold increase from 15 centers in 2012. Focusing solely on people with SMIs, these institutions can expand mental health services to psychiatric rehabilitation support. However, only 1.5 percent of the total population with SMIs requiring social assistance is served by psychiatric institutions. Although most of these individuals live in communities with minimal support (95 percent),

3.5 percent of them receive support through general SPCs (Viet Nam MOLISA 2021). Moreover, there is wide variation in rehabilitation services for individuals with SMIs across centers, depending on institutional capacity and mobilized resources (Nguyen et al. 2018). Pharmacological interventions and psychotherapies are largely unavailable for individuals with SMIs in SPCs (RTCCD 2014).

Access to institution-based social care and support remains limited in the disadvantaged regions. Given the unequal distribution of SPCs and psychiatric rehabilitation centers across the provinces, there is substantial geographic variation in access to institutional care, as visualized in map 2.1 and figure 2.3. While the Northern Upland region accommodates only 2 percent of individuals with SMIs in social welfare facilities, the Southeast region hosts close to 15 percent. Although the Central Highlands region hosts more than 5 percent of the individuals with SMIs in social welfare centers, the region has no psychiatric rehabilitation facilities.

There is also concern about the rights of people with SMIs in SPCs. Patients are often treated in therapy spaces without sufficient recreational areas, although the policy requires separate living quarters, kitchens, work areas, and recreational areas in centers with more than 25 clients (Nguyen et al. 2018). Confinement over extended periods is sometimes applied to people exhibiting aggressive behaviors due to mental illness (Nguyen, Tran, Green, et al. 2019). In recent years, significant media coverage has highlighted the conditions of treatment of individuals with SMIs in SPCs. Subsequently, the need for improvement has been put on the agenda for SPCs.

Maintaining essential services for people with SMIs is challenging for many SPCs and psychiatric rehabilitation centers. The patients, who are most often individuals with schizophrenia living in government funded institutions, receive monthly cash assistance of 450,000 VND (approximately US$20), financial

FIGURE 2.3

**Percentage of people with SMIs staying in psychiatric rehabilitation centers and SPCs across regions in Viet Nam, 2021**

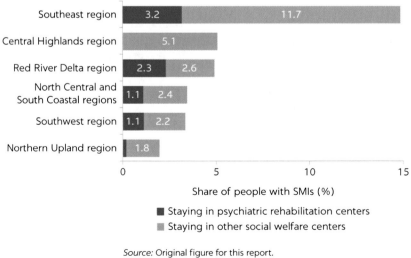

Source: Original figure for this report.
Note: SMIs = serious mental illnesses; SPC = social protection center.

support for medication, and daily life necessities, including food and clothing (Nguyen et al. 2018). Social welfare centers spend nearly three-quarters of their annual budget on food and staff salaries (Viet Nam MOLISA 2021). Consequently, medical staff often receive low wages for increasing workloads, making it difficult to retain staff (Nguyen et al. 2018).

## Community-based care and rehabilitation for individuals with mental disorders

The social sector is implementing the national program on community-based rehabilitation and social assistance for people with mental disorders. The first phase of the program (2011–20) created a foundation for community-based service delivery. It strengthened the policy framework and institutional capacities and developed the community-based rehabilitation workforce. Additionally, the first phase focused on piloting treatment models and scaling up the prevention of mental health issues by raising community awareness and participation. The second phase (2021–30) is continuing to develop more inclusive and comprehensive treatment approaches. It aims to expand the beneficiaries beyond people with SMIs to people with depression and children with ASD. Community-based rehabilitation and social assistance require collaboration across the health, education, finance, legal, and social sectors, and all 63 cities and provinces have an implementation plan with an intersectoral arrangement.

It has been challenging for the social affairs authorities to coordinate implementation of the program toward achieving the intersectoral targets. Interventions and targets related to early detection, counseling, psychotherapy, education, and family care for children who have ASD and depression require critical contributions from the health and education sectors. Within the social sector, intensive efforts are needed to deliver counseling, case management, occupational therapy, vocational guidance, livelihood support, and cultural and physical activities for people with mental disorders, in addition to public communication, monitoring, and evaluation.

The social affairs authorities rely on the social welfare network to deliver community-based rehabilitation and social assistance for people with mental disorders. Of the country's 63 cities and provinces, 36 have established provincial social work centers whose mandate includes providing vulnerable groups and victims of violence counseling, psychotherapies, and social assistance (Viet Nam MOLISA 2021). The social work centers in Ho Chi Minh City, Da Nang, and Quang Ninh, Thanh Hoa, Long An, and Ben Tre provinces offer various psychosocial services, such as psychological counseling, psychotherapy, and educational therapy, for people with mental disorders in the communities. Among the hundreds of SPCs and Psychiatric Rehabilitation Centers serving people with SMIs, several institutions in Son La, Thai Nguyen, Hai Duong, and Thua Thien Hue provinces provide a combination of occupational therapy, rotating rehabilitation schemes, and social work to improve functional recovery (Viet Nam MOLISA 2018). In addition to the provincial systems, the National Hotline for Child Protection 111 has provided 24/7 and free-of-charge counseling services for nearly 19,000 cases related to psychological problems in children (Hotline 111 2021).

Despite the presence of demonstration models in a dozen locations, the social welfare institutions have inadequate capacity to deliver services for people with mental disorders in the communities. Apart from budget constraints, many welfare institutions lack a competent workforce: each institution has only 28 staff on average, and more than 80 percent of the staff has no educational background in social work or health care (Viet Nam MOLISA 2021). Such limited capacity hinders welfare institutions from providing professional services and making greater efforts to reach potential service users in their communities.

There are limited rehabilitation and social services for people with mental disorders in rural communities. Questions about accessibility have been raised since almost all the social work centers have been established at the provincial level rather than the district level as was initially envisaged in the national plans (Viet Nam MOLISA and UNICEF 2014).[3] People with SMIs in rural areas can receive only limited assistance from commune social workers and social collaborators, whose competencies in mental health rehabilitation remain a concern. In the absence of effective rehabilitation and social services at the community level, the burden of care is placed on family members and relatives (Kidd et al. 2016), amounting to a financial loss of US$450 per year per family (Nguyen, Tran, Tran, et al. 2019). Unequal access to both health care and social assistance may contribute to the urban-rural disparity in mental health outcomes: the rates of psychiatric disabilities in rural areas are higher than those in urban areas among the adult population (1.02 versus 0.62 percent) and among children ages 5 to 17 years (2.41 versus 1.82 percent) (Viet Nam GSO 2016).

Private sector participation in care and rehabilitation for people with mental disorders is limited. Among 533 social welfare institutions nationwide, the private sector established and operates 241 centers (45.2 percent). Although it invests extensively in social welfare for children, older people, and people with disabilities, the private sector participates minimally in the care and rehabilitation of people with mental illnesses (figure 2.4).

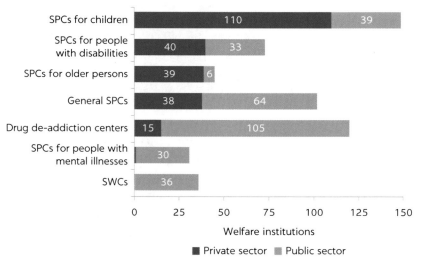

FIGURE 2.4

**Public and private welfare institutions in Viet Nam's social sector, 2021**

*Source:* Viet Nam MOLISA 2021.
*Note:* SPC = social protection center; SWC = social work center.

### Drug addiction treatment network

In addition to the health care and social welfare networks, 120 drug addiction treatment centers have been established and are in operation nationwide. They include 79 centers offering combined compulsory and voluntary treatment schemes and services, six centers offering compulsory treatment schemes, 18 centers offering voluntary treatment services, and two welfare centers for drug abusers. In 2019, these facilities provided institutional treatment to nearly 36,000 drug abusers. Among those individuals, 76.8 percent were treated under the compulsory scheme, 19.2 percent under the voluntary arrangement, and 4 percent under the welfare scheme (Viet Nam MOLISA 2021). Reported problems at these institutional facilities include overloaded infrastructure in the compulsory treatment centers, unsatisfactory living conditions, limited psychotherapies and behavioral therapies, and insufficient competencies among the employees (Viet Nam MOLISA 2021).

Community-based addiction treatment and support services are available in selected cities and provinces. In 2013, the government adopted a new drug addiction treatment strategy, which expanded the treatment network to the community level.[4] Around 800 community-based sites have been established in 23 cities and provinces to provide care, counseling, and treatment support for drug abusers. These sites are mainly integrated into CHSs and supported by a commune de-addiction task force. The task force's scope of work includes detection of patients with addictions and evaluation of their circumstances; provision of counseling and registration for treatment schemes; monitoring and supervision of individuals with addiction disorders; preparation of drug user profiles; and provision of social assistance for vocational learning, job seeking, and community integration. Nevertheless, pressing issues related to recovery support remain, as addiction, relapse, and unemployment are common among drug users in the communities.

The private sector has invested significantly in drug addiction treatment facilities since the government encourages voluntary de-addiction services. In 2015, 22 private drug addiction treatment centers were established countrywide (Viet Nam MOLISA 2021). However, the private investment momentum was not maintained due to weak demand from individuals with drug addictions. At least seven private centers have been closed over the past five years.

## MENTAL HEALTH SERVICES IN THE EDUCATION SECTOR

Education policy makers have realized and responded to the increasing need for care and education for children and adolescents with mental disorders. Thanks to inclusive education policies, 94.2 percent of students with disabilities, including intellectual and mental ones, were educated in general classes (Hai 2020) and 72.8 percent of children with ASD were learning in inclusive education settings rather than special education institutions (Tran, Pham, et al. 2020). To ensure students' access to mental health services, the Ministry of Education and Training requested all schools to create a health office with a health worker,[5] establish a psychological counseling group,[6] and ensure that all the students have universal health insurance coverage.[7] The national school health program[8] aims to provide mental health communication and counseling to 50 percent of the students by 2025.

However, most schools in Viet Nam, like those in other low- and middle-income countries, have limited resources to address mental health issues in line with the national guidelines. Only 50 percent of schools have a health office, and only 40 percent of school health personnel meet the required professional qualifications (*People Newspaper* 2020). Given the shortage of professional psychological counselors, schools have appointed teachers to form psychological counseling groups, but they lack expertise in this area. It was estimated that 70,000 teachers countrywide would need to be trained in psychological counseling to fill the competency gap (*Vietnam News* 2018).

Although almost all students are insured for access to care, school-based mental health services remain largely unavailable or insufficient. Adolescents in secondary and high schools prefer seeking help from friends, relatives, or family members rather than teachers and school counselors (Thai, Vu, and Bui 2020). University students exhibiting symptoms of anxiety and depression commonly utilize mental health services at hospitals and clinics outside their campus (Nam et al. 2021). Explicit stigmatization of mental illness may prevent students from seeking help from teachers and using school-based services. Several school-based mental health interventions have been implemented; however, these small-scale projects are fragmented across the country's different regions (Tran, Nguyen, et al. 2020).

Schools and teachers have encountered many difficulties in providing inclusive education for students with mental disorders. The main challenges that schools face are budget constraints and lack of expertise. Eighty-six percent of schools reported that they had no budget allocation for educating children with disabilities, 86 percent had no access to a disability adviser, and 95 percent did not have a disability specialist (UNICEF 2015). Although ASD was recognized as a neurodevelopmental disorder,[9] preschool teachers have fundamental misconceptions about the cause, diagnosis, and treatment of ASD (Vu and Tran 2014). Teachers face significant problems, including limited access to educational curricula, inadequate teaching aids, and inexperience in child behavior management, which hinder them from providing effective education for children with ASD in general education classrooms (Van Tran et al. 2020).

There is encouraging participation from the private sector in the care and education of children with mental illnesses, although service quality remains a concern. Over the past decade, more than 60 private facilities have been established in 19 cities and provinces (Tran and Weiss 2018), which has improved accessibility to early identification and intervention services for children with ASD. Although there have been improvements in mental health service provision, studies also raise questions about the quality of care, suggesting that a significant number of care providers do not have the appropriate legal status and do not follow basic ethical standards and evidence-based intervention methods (Tran and Weiss 2018; Tran et al. 2015). An oversight mechanism is needed to ensure effective and sustainable engagement of the private sector in the care and education of children with mental disorders.

## INFORMAL CAREGIVERS FOR PEOPLE WITH MENTAL DISORDERS

Informal services are provided by nonprofessional people who do not work in formal mental health systems. Informal caregivers include family members, relatives, friends, traditional healers, village health workers, social collaborators, teachers, peer support groups, other community members, and even people with mental disorders themselves. Informal services are necessary, and they are even more critical for individuals with SMIs, as 95 percent of them live in their communities.

Family care plays a vital role in mental health care, and family members directly influence health-seeking behaviors and access to health care services. Nearly 80 percent of people with SMIs are cared for by family members such as their parents, spouse, or children (RTCCD 2014). However, due to the lack of professional support, the quality of family care could be improved. Nearly 40 percent of people with SMIs who are staying at home receive neither treatment nor entertainment support (RTCCD 2014).

People with mental disorders and family members often seek help from informal community caregivers. Traditional healing is widely accepted in Vietnamese society and offers various medicinal herbs, acupuncture, acupressure, massage, qigong, and so forth, and spiritual healing is common. Depending on the respective religious affiliation, Buddhist pagodas and Christian churches play an important role in helping people with mental health problems by providing spiritual counseling. This includes the Buddhist practices of mindfulness and meditation, community belonging, interpretation of lessons from life philosophy, religious stories, and chanting or performing rituals (Nguyen 2013, 2014, 2016). With the development of social networks and online communities, peer support groups are increasing at a remarkable rate, among which peer-to-peer support for parents of children with ASD has become especially popular.

People with mental disorders often play a passive role in self-managing their mental illness. Mental health literacy among the general population needs to improve, to enable people to recognize symptoms and seek appropriate help at an early stage (Dang et al. 2020; Nguyen, Tran, Green, et al. 2019; Thai, Vu, and Bui 2020). People with SMIs have little voice and choice in institutional care and treatment (Nguyen, Tran, Green, et al. 2019). Furthermore, there is limited understanding and promotion of self-care in Viet Nam. However, self-care and basic mental health literacy build the foundation for a functioning mental health care system (WHO and World Organization of Family Doctors 2008).

## NOTES

1. Ministry of Health Circular No. 39/2017/TT-BYT, dated October 18, 2017, regulated the primary health service package for the grassroots level.
2. Prime Minister Decision No. 1125/QĐ-TTg, dated July 31, 2018, approved the Viet Nam Health–Population Program 2016–20.
3. Prime Minister Decision No. 32/2010/QĐ-TTg, dated March 25, 2010, and Inter-Ministerial Circular 09/2013/TTLT-BLĐTBXH-BNV, dated June 10, 2013, regulated the organization of social work centers.
4. Prime Minister Decision 2596/QĐ-TTg, dated December 27, 2013, approved the drug de-addiction reform project until 2020.
5. Inter-Circular No. 13/2016/TTLT-BYT-BGDĐT, dated May 12, 2016, regulated school health services.
6. Ministry of Education and Training Circular No. 31/2017/TT-BGDĐT, dated December 18, 2017, regulated school psychological counseling services.
7. Government's Decree 146/2018/NĐ-CP, dated October 17, 2018, regulated and guided the implementation of the Health Issuance Law.
8. Prime Minister Decision 1660/QĐ-TTg, dated October 2, 2021, approved the school health program 2021–2025.
9. Ministry of Education and Training Official Letter No. 9771/BGDĐT – HSSV, dated October 28, 2005, guided the implementation of counseling for students.

## REFERENCES

Babalola, E., N. Pia, and W. Ross. 2017. "The Biopsychosocial Approach and Global Mental Health: Synergies and Opportunities." *Indian Journal of Social Psychiatry* 33 (4): 291–96.

Boardman, J., and S. Dave. 2020. "Person-Centred Care and Psychiatry: Some Key Perspectives." *BJPsych International* 17 (3): 65–68.

Böge, K., E. Hahn, T. D. Cao, L. M. Fuchs, L. K. Martensen, G. Schomerus, M. Dettling, M. Angermeyer, V. T. Nguyen, and T. M. T. Ta. 2018. "Treatment Recommendation Differences for Schizophrenia and Major Depression: A Population-Based Study in a Vietnamese Cohort." *International Journal of Mental Health Systems* 12 (1): 1–11.

CEHS (Center for Environmental Health Study). 2020. "Evaluation of Primary Healthcare Teams' Post-Training Performance under the Health Professional Education and Training for Health System Reforms Project." CEHS, Hanoi.

Cuong, T. V. 2017. "Mental Health Care in Vietnam." *American Journal of Psychiatry* 31: 287.

Dang, H. M., T. T. Lam, A. Dao, and B. Weiss. 2020. "Mental Health Literacy at the Public Health Level in Low and Middle Income Countries: An Exploratory Mixed Methods Study in Vietnam." *PLoS One* 15 (12): e0244573. https://doi.org/10.1371/journal.pone.0244573.

Do, M. T., T. T. Nguyen, and H. T. T. Tran. 2022. "Preliminary Results of Adapting the Stepped Care Model for Depression Management in Vietnam." *Frontiers in Psychiatry* 13: 922911. https://doi.org/10.3389/fpsyt.2022.922911.

Go, D.-S., K.-C. Shin, J.-W. Paik, K.-A. Kim, and S.-J. Yoon. 2020. "A Review of the Admission System for Mental Disorders in South Korea." *International Journal of Environmental Research and Public Health* 17 (24): 9159.

Hai, N. X. 2020. "Sustainable Development of Inclusive Education for Persons with Disabilities in Vietnam." *International Journal of Asian Social Science* 10 (12): 761–70.

Hotline 111. 2021. "Achievements of the National Hotline 111 for National Child Protection since Its Establishment." Hotline 111 (accessed October 13, 2021), http://tongdai111.vn/tin/et-qua-hoat-dong-cua-tong-dai-quoc-gia-bao-ve-tre-em-111-tu-khi-van-hanh-den-nay.

Humphries, S. H., R. J. King, M. P. Dunne, and N. H. Cat. 2015. "Psychiatrists' Perceptions of What Determines Outcomes for People Diagnosed with Schizophrenia in Vietnam." *ASEAN Journal of Psychiatry* 16 (2): 181–92.

Khue, P. M., N. T. Tham, D. T. Thanh Mai, P. V. Thuc, V. M. Thuc, P. V. Han, and C. Lindan. 2017. "A Longitudinal and Case-Control Study of Dropout among Drug Users in Methadone Maintenance Treatment in Haiphong, Vietnam." *Harm Reduction Journal* 14 (1): 59. https://doi.org/10.1186/s12954-017-0185-7.

Kidd, S., T. Abu-el-Haj, B. Khondker, C. Watson, and S. Ramkissoon. 2016. *Social Assistance in Viet Nam: A Review and Proposals for Reform.* Hanoi: Development Pathways and United Nations Development Programme.

McCance-Katz, E. F. 2018. "The Substance Abuse and Mental Health Services Administration (SAMHSA): New Directions." *Psychiatric Services* 69 (10, October). https://doi.org/10.1176/appi.ps.201800281.

Minas, H., and M. Lewis. 2017. *Mental Health in Asia and the Pacific: Historical and Cultural Perspectives.* New York: Springer.

Nam, P. T., P. T. Tung, D. Nguyen Hanh, D. H. An, A. Bui Dang The, G. Kim Bao, G. Dang Huong, H. N. Thi Thu, H. Pham Ngoc, and H. Nguyen Thi Thanh. 2021. "Utilization of Mental Health Services among University Students in Vietnam." *International Journal of Mental Health* 50 (2): 113–35.

Ng, C. H., P. T. Than, C. D. La, Q. Van Than, and C. Van Dieu. 2011a. "The National Community Mental Health Care Project in Vietnam: A Review for Future Guidance." *Australasian Psychiatry* 19 (2): 143–50.

Ng, C. H., P. T. Than, C. D. La, Q. Van Than, and C. Van Dieu. 2011b. "Outcomes and Future Directions of the National Community Mental Health Care Program in Viet Nam." *World Psychiatry* 10 (2): 153.

Ngo, V. K., B. Weiss, T. Lam, T. Dang, T. Nguyen, and M. H. Nguyen. 2014. "The Vietnam Multicomponent Collaborative Care for Depression Program: Development of Depression Care for Low- and Middle-Income Nations." *Journal of Cognitive Psychotherapy* 28 (3): 156–67.

Nguyen, H. 2013. "Linking Social Work with Buddhist Temples: Developing a Model of Mental Health Service Delivery and Treatment in Vietnam." *British Journal of Social Work* 45 (4): 1242–58. https://doi.org/10.1093/bjsw/bct181.

Nguyen, H. 2014. "Buddhism-Based Exorcism and Spirit-Calling as a Form of Healing for People with Mental Health Problems: Stories from Vietnam." *Journal of Social Work in Religion and Spirituality* 33 (1): 33–48. https://doi.org/10.1080/15426432.2014.873648.

Nguyen, H. 2016. "Mental Health Care for Elderly People at Formal Mental Health Systems and Buddhist Temples in Vietnam: Making a Case for Mindful Elder Care in Vietnam." *Ageing International* 41 (4): 394–413. https://doi.org/10.1007/s12126-016-9263-5.

Nguyen, H. V., H. T. H. Do, V. T. A. Le, and N.-A. Mai. 2018. "Reviewing the Latest National Policies and Services for People with Severe Mental Health Disorders in Government-Funded Institutions in Vietnam and Policy Recommendations for Service Improvements." *Asia Pacific Journal of Social Work and Development* 28 (1): 56–68.

Nguyen, T., T. Tran, S. Green, A. Hsueh, T. Tran, H. Tran, and J. Fisher. 2019. "Delays to Diagnosis among People with Severe Mental Illness in Rural Vietnam: A Population-Based Cross-Sectional Survey." *BMC Psychiatry* 19 (1): 1–11.

Nguyen, T., T. Tran, H. Tran, T. Tran, and J. Fisher. 2019. "Challenges in Integrating Mental Health into Primary Care in Vietnam." In *Innovations in Global Mental Health*, edited by S. Okpaku, 1–21. Cham, Switzerland: Springer International Publishing. http://doi.org/10.1007/978-3-319-70134-9_74-1.

Nguyen, T., T. Tran, S. Green, et al. 2020. "Proof of Concept of Participant Informed, Psycho-Educational, Community-Based Intervention for People with Severe Mental Illness in Rural Vietnam." *International Journal of Social Psychiatry* 66 (3): 232–39. https://doi.org/10.1177/0020764019898234.

Niemi, M. S. Kiel, P. Allebeck, and L. T. Hoan. 2016. "Community-Based Intervention for Depression Management at the Primary Care Level in Ha Nam Province, Vietnam: A Cluster-Randomized Controlled Trial." *Tropical Medicine and International Health* 21 (5): 654–61. https://doi.org/:10.1111/tmi.12674.

OECD (Organisation for Economic Co-operation and Development). 2014. *Making Mental Health Count.* https://www.oecd.org/els/health-systems/Focus-on-Health-Making-Mental-Health-Count.pdf.

*People Newspaper.* 2020. "Paying Adequate Attention to School Health." *People Newspaper*, Hanoi (accessed October 16, 2021), https://nhandan.vn/baothoinay-xahoi/quan-tam-thich-dang-y-te-hoc-duong-579948?fbclid=IwAR1SCq07p2G4-WgoLRvLpJq3ITe-DRc4-62oZe9Pby46hRE7V6qcQsjoZ0Y.

RTCCD (Research and Training Centre for Community Development). 2014. *Baseline Survey on Mental Healthcare System for People with Mental Illness in Thanh Hoa and Ben Tre Provinces.* Hanoi, Viet Nam: RTCCD.

Thai, T. T., N. L. L. T. Vu, and H. H. T. Bui. 2020. "Mental Health Literacy and Help-Seeking Preferences in High School Students in Ho Chi Minh City, Vietnam." *School Mental Health* 12 (2): 378–87.

Tran, C. V., M. M. Pham, P. T. Mai, T. T. Le, and D. T. Nguyen. 2020. "Inclusive Education for Students with Autism Spectrum Disorder in Elementary Schools in Vietnam: The Current Situation and Solutions." *International Electronic Journal of Elementary Education* 12 (3): 265–73.

Tran, C. V., and B. Weiss. 2018. "Characteristics of Agencies Providing Support Services for Children with Autism Spectrum Disorders in Vietnam." *International Journal of Social Science and Humanity* 8 (4): 116.

Tran, C. V., B. Weiss, T. N. Khuc, T. T. L. Tran, T. T. N. Nguyen, H. T. K. Nguyen, and T. T. T. Dao. 2015. "Early Identification and Intervention Services for Children with Autism in Vietnam." *Health Psychology Report* 3 (3): 191–200. https://doi.org/10.5114/hpr.2015.53125.

Tran, T., H. T. Nguyen, I. Shochet, A. Wurfl, J. Orr, N. Nguyen, N. La, et al. 2020. "School-Based, Two-Arm, Parallel, Controlled Trial of a Culturally Adapted Resilience Intervention to Improve Adolescent Mental Health in Vietnam: Study Protocol." *BMJ Open* 10 (10): e039343. https://doi.org/10.1136/bmjopen-2020-039343.

Tran, T., B. La, and T. Nguyen. 2007. *Evaluation of National Community Mental Health Care Project.* Hanoi: Viet Nam Research and Training Center for Community Development.

UNICEF (United Nations Children's Fund). 2015. *Readiness for the Education of Children with Disabilities in Eight Provinces of Vietnam.* Hanoi: UNICEF Viet Nam.

Van, N. H. N., N. Thi Khanh Huyen, M. T. Hue, N. T. Luong, P. Quoc Thanh, D. M. Duc, V. Thi Thanh Mai, and T. T. Hong. 2021. "Perceived Barriers to Mental Health Services among the Elderly in the Rural of Vietnam: A Cross-Sectional Survey in 2019." *Health Services Insights* 14: 11786329211026035.

Van Tran, C., M. M. Pham, P. T. Mai, T. T. Le, and D. T. Nguyen. 2020. "Inclusive Education for Students with Autism Spectrum Disorder in Elementary Schools in Vietnam: The Current Situation and Solutions." *International Electronic Journal of Elementary Education* 12 (3): 265–73.

Viet Nam GSO (General Statistics Office of Viet Nam). 2016. *The National Survey on People with Disabilities 2016.* VDS2016 Final Report. Hanoi: Viet Nam GSO.

Viet Nam MOH (Ministry of Health of Viet Nam). 2018. *The Program Targeting Health–Population Program 2016–2020: New Features in Fund Management and Utilization.* Hanoi: Viet Nam MOH.

Viet Nam MOH (Ministry of Health of Viet Nam). 2019. *Health Statistics Yearbook 2017–2018.* Hanoi: Medical Publishing House.

Viet Nam MOH (Ministry of Health of Viet Nam). 2020. "An Online Forum on Digital Remedies for Strengthening Non-Communicable Disease Care and Treatment in the New Normal." September 22, Viet Nam MOH, Hanoi.

Viet Nam MOH (Ministry of Health of Viet Nam). 2023. *Draft Proposal for Mental Health System Strengthening.* Hanoi: Viet Nam MOH.

Viet Nam MOLISA (Ministry of Labour, Invalids, and Social Affairs of Viet Nam). 2018. *Evaluation Report: The Implementation of the Legal Framework on Social Work.* Hanoi: Viet Nam MOLISA.

Viet Nam MOLISA (Ministry of Labour, Invalids, and Social Affairs of Viet Nam). 2021. *Draft Master Plan for the Social Welfare Network in the Period of 2021–2030 with a Vision to 2050.* Hanoi: Viet Nam MOLISA.

Viet Nam MOLISA and UNICEF (Ministry of Labour, Invalids, and Social Affairs of Viet Nam and United Nations Children's Fund). 2014. "Review of the Implementation of Decision 32/2010/QĐ-TTg Concerning National Plan 32 to Develop Professional Social Work." In *Report of the Progress Review Conducted by the Ministry of Labour, Invalids and Social Affairs with UNICEF Viet Nam.* Hanoi: Viet Nam MOLISA and UNICEF.

*Vietnam News.* 2018. "Students' Mental Health Should Be a Focus." *Vietnam News,* April 28. https://vietnamnews.vn/society/427029/students-mental-health-should-be-a-focus.html.

Vu, T. V., and C. V. Tran. 2014. "Attitude of Preschool Teachers in Hanoi on Autism Spectrum Disorders." *Proceedings of the National Mental Health in Schools Conference,* 486–96.

WHO (World Health Organization). 2019. *The Global Health Observatory: Explore a World of Health Data.* Geneva: WHO. https://www.who.int/data/gho/data/themes/topics/indicator-groups/indicator-group-details/GHO/beds.

WHO (World Health Organization). 2021. *Mental Health Atlas 2020.* Geneva: WHO.

WHO and Viet Nam MOH (World Health Organization and Ministry of Health of Viet Nam). 2006. *WHO-AIMS Report on Mental Health System in Vietnam.* Geneva: WHO.

WHO and World Organization of Family Doctors. 2008. *Integrating Mental Health into Primary Care: A Global Perspective.* Geneva: WHO.

World Bank. 2019. *Vietnam National and Provincial Primary Health Care Scorecards.* Washington, DC: World Bank.

Xia, L., F. Jiang, J. Rakofsky, Y. Zhang, Y. Shi, K. Zhang, T. Liu, Y. Liu, H. Liu, and Y.-I. Tang. 2021. "Resources and Workforce in Top-Tier Psychiatric Hospitals in China: A Nationwide Survey." *Frontiers in Psychiatry* 12. https://doi.org/10.3389/fpsyt.2021.573333.

# 3 Mental Health Workforce in Viet Nam

## INTRODUCTION

This chapter describes the current situation of the mental health workforce in Viet Nam. It analyzes critical issues, including the shortage of professionals and their numbers (psychiatrists, mental health nurses, psychologists, social workers, and others), maldistribution between levels and regions, competency mismatch, job dissatisfaction, recruitment, and retention issues.

## TYPES OF MENTAL HEALTH PROFESSIONALS IN VIET NAM

In this study, mental health professionals include those who work in the formal sectors (health, social, education, and community-based organizations) and provide care and support to people with mental disorders. Table 3.1 summarizes the types of mental health professionals whose professional identity is recognized by the government of Viet Nam.

## PSYCHIATRISTS AND MENTAL HEALTH DOCTORS

Viet Nam has been suffering from a persistent shortage of psychiatrists. An estimated 609 psychiatrists—medical doctors by training with at least two years of postgraduate training in psychiatry—were working in Viet Nam in 2021. They were employed by central psychiatric hospitals (26.1 percent), provincial psychiatric hospitals (66.0 percent), psychiatric units in general hospitals (5.4 percent), and mental health units in provincial Centers for Disease Control (CDCs) (2.5 percent). The ratio of psychiatrists per 100,000 population reached 0.62 in 2021, which was higher than the average for low- and lower-middle-income countries (0.40) but far below the global average (1.70) (WHO 2021) (figure 3.1).

In 2021, mental health care facilities in Viet Nam employed 557 mental health doctors—medical doctors with fewer than two years of postgraduate training in psychiatry. Mental health doctors work in provincial psychiatric hospitals (83.0 percent), central psychiatric hospitals (9.5 percent), psychiatric units in

TABLE 3.1 **Formal mental health professionals in Viet Nam**

| PROFESSIONALS | SECTOR | WORKPLACES | MENTAL HEALTH SERVICES |
|---|---|---|---|
| Psychiatrists | Health | Psychiatric hospitals and psychiatric wards | Assessment, diagnosis, treatment, and care at the specialized level |
| Mental health doctors | | | |
| Mental health nurses | Health | Psychiatric hospitals and psychiatric wards | Screening, assessment, and care at the specialized level |
| Psychologists | Social, health, and education | Counseling centers, social welfare centers, hospitals, and schools | Prevention, promotion, screening, assessment, counseling, and psychotherapy |
| Social service workers | Social and health | Social welfare centers, hospitals, and community-based organizations | Prevention, promotion, screening, and social assistance in recovery |

*Source:* Original table for this report.

FIGURE 3.1

**Psychiatrists per 100,000 population in Viet Nam and other countries, by World Bank income group, 2021**

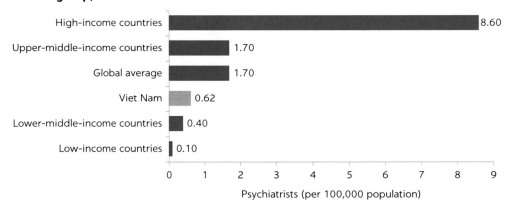

*Source:* Original figure for this report based on World Health Organization data.

general hospitals (3.9 percent), and mental health units in provincial CDCs (3.6 percent). In the disadvantaged provinces, mental health doctors were the main providers of mental illness diagnoses and psychopharmaceutical treatments.

The engagement of medical doctors in mental health care has resulted in a growing and young psychiatry workforce. Between 2004 and 2021, the number of psychiatrists in Viet Nam more than doubled, from 286 to 609, and the ratio of psychiatrists per 100,000 population increased from 0.35 to 0.62 (based on data from WHO and Viet Nam MOH (2006) and the survey for this study). From 2016 to 2020, mental health care facilities nationwide recruited 272 new medical doctors and pensioned 158 others. Additionally, each year, the psychiatry education system supplements the workforce with 25 to 30 new psychiatrists who have completed a psychiatry residency program or a psychiatry specialist program. By 2021, an estimated 1.2 percent of all medical doctors in the country had selected a career in psychiatry. As a result, Viet Nam has a young psychiatry workforce, in which 72.6 percent of the psychiatrists and mental health doctors are younger than 50 years and only 4.9 percent are at retirement age (60 or older).

However, access to a psychiatrist or mental health doctor varies across geo-economic regions. The median number of psychiatrists is 10 times higher in the Red River Delta region (1.14 psychiatrists per 100,000 population) than in the Central Highlands region (0.12) and 3.5 times higher than in the Southwest region (0.32) (figure 3.2). The disparity is also evident between cities and provinces in different income groups, ranging from 0.17 psychiatrist per 100,000 population in the 10 lowest-income provinces to 1.13 psychiatrists per 100,000 population in the 10 highest-income cities and provinces.

Furthermore, the psychiatry workforce in Viet Nam is highly urbanized. In all localities, the psychiatrists are employed by central- and provincial-level facilities; therefore, they are concentrated in urban areas with limited outreach services to rural communities. Employment of mental health doctors would mitigate the severe shortage of psychiatrists in the disadvantaged provinces, but it would not narrow the urban-rural divide (map 3.1).

Even in medium-size and small cities, recruitment for the mental health workforce is a significant concern. Between 2016 and 2020, mental health care facilities in provincial-level cities recruited 151 medical doctors, achieving only 32 percent of their recruitment plans. In 2020, more than half of the provinces reported that they did not recruit any new psychiatrists. In contrast, psychiatric hospitals and psychiatric units in large cities, like Hanoi and Ho Chi Minh City, attracted more medical doctors than expected, achieving 175 percent of their recruitment targets (figure 3.3).

Because their working conditions are unfavorable, most psychiatrists and mental health doctors are only somewhat satisfied with many aspects of their jobs. Public attitudes toward psychiatrists are negative (Ta et al. 2018). As 92 percent of mental health doctors report that their income is less than 10 million VND (equivalent to US$430) per month, compensation packages are less competitive in psychiatry than in other medical professions. Fringe benefits,

FIGURE 3.2

**Psychiatrists and mental health doctors per 100,000 population in Viet Nam, by geo-economic region, 2021**

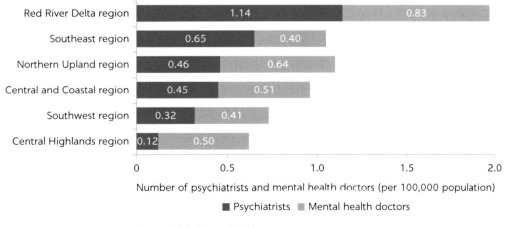

*Source:* Original figure for this report.

MAP 3.1
**Distribution of psychiatrists in Viet Nam mainland, 2021**

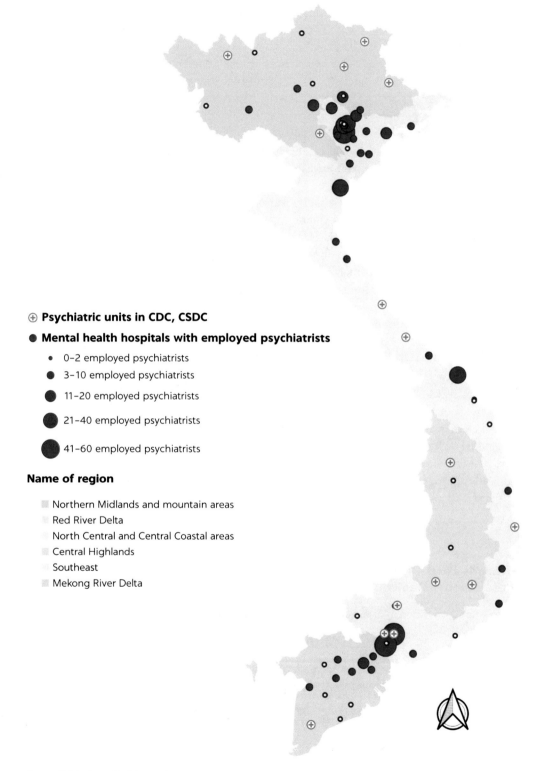

⊕ **Psychiatric units in CDC, CSDC**

● **Mental health hospitals with employed psychiatrists**

- · 0–2 employed psychiatrists
- ● 3–10 employed psychiatrists
- ● 11–20 employed psychiatrists
- ● 21–40 employed psychiatrists
- ● 41–60 employed psychiatrists

**Name of region**

- ▨ Northern Midlands and mountain areas
- ▨ Red River Delta
- ▨ North Central and Central Coastal areas
- ▨ Central Highlands
- ▨ Southeast
- ▨ Mekong River Delta

*Source:* Original map for this report.
*Note:* CDC = Centers for Disease Control; CSDC = Centers for Social Disease Control.

FIGURE 3.3

**Mental health care facilities' planned and actual recruitment of medical doctors, 2016–20**

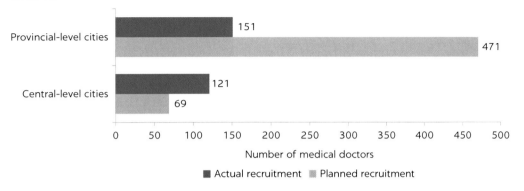

*Source:* Original figure for this report.

FIGURE 3.4

**Job satisfaction of psychiatrists and mental health doctors, 2021**

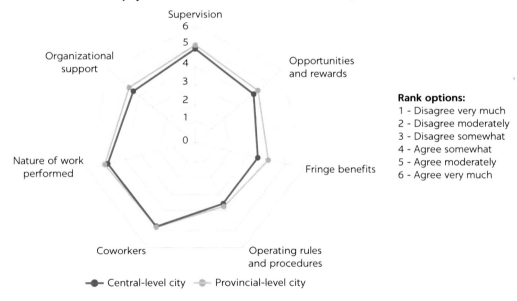

**Rank options:**
1 - Disagree very much
2 - Disagree moderately
3 - Disagree somewhat
4 - Agree somewhat
5 - Agree moderately
6 - Agree very much

*Source:* Original figure for this report.
*Note:* The figure shows the level of job satisfaction by category, on a scale from 1 to 6 (very unsatisfied to very satisfied).

opportunities and rewards, and operating rules and procedures are the three main areas of job dissatisfaction, particularly among young professionals receiving low salaries and those working in large cities (figure 3.4). The level of job satisfaction among psychiatrists and mental health doctors increases with age and income (figure 3.5).

FIGURE 3.5

**Job satisfaction, average income, and years on the job of psychiatrists and mental health doctors, 2021**

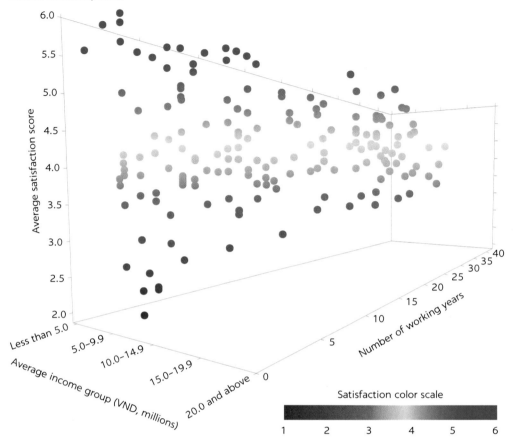

Source: Original figure for this report.
Note: The figure shows the level of job satisfaction by category, on a scale from 1 to 6 (very unsatisfied to very satisfied).

## MENTAL HEALTH NURSES

Like the psychiatry workforce, the mental health nursing workforce is growing. As of 2020, Viet Nam had three mental health nurses per 100,000 population, which was higher than the average for low- and lower-middle-income countries and close to the global average (figure 3.6). Almost all the mental health nurses provide institutional care in provincial psychiatric hospitals (75.0 percent), central psychiatric hospitals (19.8 percent), and psychiatric units in general hospitals (4.4 percent). Only 0.8 percent of the mental health nurses worked in mental health units in provincial CDCs.

Increased recruitment of nurses into mental health facilities has contributed significantly to workforce growth. Between 2016 and 2020, mental health care facilities nationwide newly recruited 673 nurses and pensioned 260 others. Actual recruitment exceeded 220 percent of the planned target at the central level and reached 80 percent of the intended target at the provincial level (figure 3.7). Currently, the country has a young mental health nursing workforce, 75 percent of which is younger than 40 years.

FIGURE 3.6

**Nurses per 100,000 population in Viet Nam and other countries, by World Bank income group, 2021**

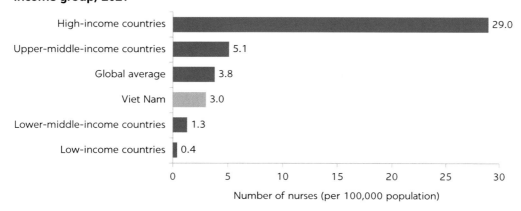

*Source:* Original figure for this report.

FIGURE 3.7

**Mental health care facilities' planned and actual recruitment of nurses, 2016–20**

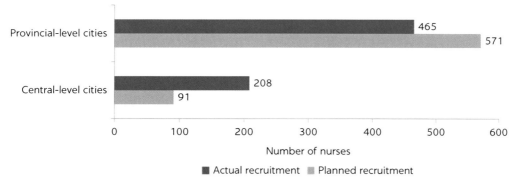

*Source:* Original figure for this report.

The mental health nursing workforce shares common features with the psychiatry workforce in terms of maldistribution and unfavorable working conditions. As they are stationed in the central and provincial hospitals, mental health nurses are concentrated in the advantaged areas. The Red River Delta region has 22 percent of the total population but employs 42 percent of the mental health nursing workforce. The ratio of mental health nurses per 100,000 population in this region (5.7) exceeds the global average (3.8). It is 2.4 times higher than that in the Southeast region (2.4), 3.2 times higher than that in the Northern Upland region (1.8), and 4.1 times higher than that in the Central Highlands region (1.4), as shown in figure 3.8.

The mental health nurses are not fully satisfied with their working conditions, as 86.7 percent of them reported a monthly income of less than 10 million VND (equivalent to US$400). In addition to fringe benefits, opportunities and rewards and operating rules and procedures are critical aspects of job dissatisfaction. Those working at the central level are less satisfied than their colleagues at the provincial level (figure 3.9).

FIGURE 3.8

**Mental health nurses per 100,000 population in Viet Nam, by geo-economic region, 2021**

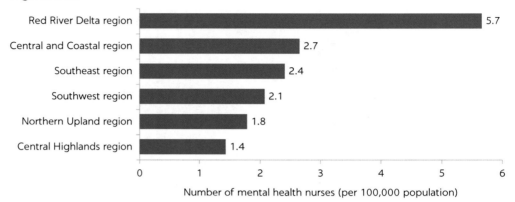

Source: Original figure for this report.

FIGURE 3.9

**Job satisfaction of mental health nurses, 2021**

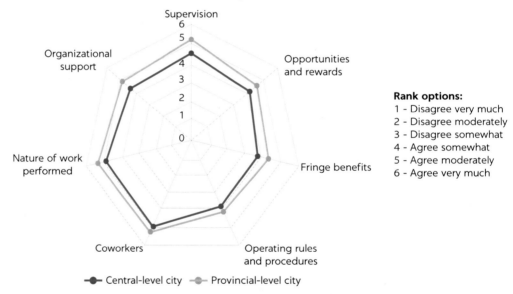

Source: Original figure for this report.
Note: The figure shows the level of job satisfaction by category, on a scale from 1 to 6 (very unsatisfied to very satisfied).

## PSYCHOLOGISTS

The psychological workforce includes clinical psychologists and psychotherapists, and school psychology counselors.

### Clinical psychologists and psychotherapists

A very small proportion of the mental health workforce in the public sector comprises psychologists and psychotherapists. There are only 143 clinical psychologists and psychotherapists (equivalent to 3 percent of clinicians) in public hospitals across Viet Nam. This means that just one psychological practitioner works with eight medical practitioners (psychiatrists and mental health doctors) and 20 nursing practitioners in clinical settings. This skill mix imbalance poses a significant challenge to operating multidisciplinary teams and delivering integrated care for patients with mental disorders. Within the residential centers for people with serious mental illnesses (SMIs), only 6.5 percent of caregivers have a background of education in psychology (Nguyen 2019).

Clinical psychologists and psychotherapists are mainly located in wealthier cities, increasing the urban-rural divide in access to mental health services. Nearly two-thirds (65.7 percent) of those who work in psychiatric hospitals are based in four cities—Hanoi, Bien Hoa, Da Nang, and Ho Chi Minh City. Meanwhile, 37 of the 63 provincial health systems have neither psychologists nor psychotherapists in public health facilities.

Although most psychologists and psychotherapists work in the private health sector, there is still unmet demand. Psychologists and psychotherapists often provide psycho-educational interventions to children with delayed language development, autism, or intellectual disability. With the growing interest in the field, psychologists are in high demand. However, most of the students who graduate with degrees in this field have limited clinical experience that does not meet the operational requirements of clinics. Therefore, early career professionals often need further training to transfer their theoretical knowledge to clinical mental health practice.

## School psychology counselors

School psychology counselors have been present in Viet Nam for two decades. The establishment of the Viet Nam Association of Psychology and Education in 2002 and the Ministry of Education and Training's guidance on school counseling in 2005 created the initial foundation for introducing psychological counselors in the education sector.[1] School managers, teachers, parents, and communities have increasingly acknowledged the importance of school psychologists for improving students' well-being, particularly during the COVID-19 pandemic. In late 2020, the government of Viet Nam recognized school psychology as a formal occupation.[2]

Despite recent developments, the professional position of school psychologist needs to be better structured in the education system. The job description, responsibilities, and salary scale for school psychologists have not been regulated. Schools often assign psychology counseling roles to existing staff and establish a psychology counseling team composed of teachers, a school health worker, and a youth union worker as guided by the Ministry of Education and Training.[3] Two-thirds of the psychology counselors concurrently hold other positions at schools, posing limitations to fulfilling their counseling tasks (Nguyen, Huynh et al. 2018). Furthermore, there are concerns about whether this arrangement ensures accountability and promotes professionalism among those who do psychology counseling as extra work. A competency framework for school psychologists to build professional credibility has been discussed, but it is yet to be concluded and approved (Le et al. 2021).

Consequently, schools nationwide lack competent psychology counselors for students. Teachers and youth union workers do not have an educational background in health sciences, and school health workers are mostly doctors' assistants and nurses with intermediate and associate degrees (Viet Nam MOH and MOET 2017). Studies show that teachers and staff who are assigned to the counselor role cannot clearly define the responsibilities of a school counselor and have not been adequately trained in some specific skills, such as substance use, HIV/AIDS counseling, crisis intervention, and grief and loss counseling (Pham 2021). Many school health workers do not know the names of specific mental illnesses, although they can recognize signs of abnormal mental health in their students.

In addition to competency mismatch, school psychology counselors encounter challenges in their working conditions. School managers often allocate unprofessionally designed rooms for psychology counseling and pay less attention to assessment activities (Nguyen, Huynh et al. 2018). In-school resources for psychology counseling are limited, and collaboration with external partners needs to be improved.[4] Furthermore, lack of recognition from parents and students is cited as another barrier to effective counseling service delivery (Pham 2021).

## SOCIAL SERVICE WORKERS

The social service workforce in Viet Nam is composed of 235,000 employees who work with vulnerable groups to ensure their well-being and development. This workforce includes 35,000 workers in social assistance networks, nearly 100,000 workers in socio-political unions, and more than 100,000 collaborators at the commune level. Although social work has evolved into a profession, other categories of paraprofessionals, such as caregivers and community collaborators, also make invaluable contributions to mental health.

### Social workers

Social workers have been positioned in the mental health system through two different frameworks. In the social sector, job positions for social work are created in all social service facilities including psychiatric care and rehabilitation centers at a quota of one social worker for every 100 managed cases.[5] In the health sector, social work teams are established in all psychiatric hospitals. The job descriptions of mental health social workers are somewhat different between the two sectors. Social workers in psychiatric care and rehabilitation centers should be patient-focused, with social work services and case management; the tasks of those in psychiatric hospitals extend to the areas of information, communication, education, training, and stakeholder engagement.[6]

Qualification-employment mismatch is a challenge facing social workers, particularly in the mental health domain. Only 12 percent of human resources in psychiatric care and rehabilitation centers have a social work degree (Nguyen 2019), and 86.5 percent of social work personnel in hospitals and 81.5 percent of those in social service facilities do not have any educational background in social work (HUPH 2019; Viet Nam MOLISA 2021). In the survey for this study, only 30 social work professionals were employed in mental health care facilities nationwide, accounting for 0.5 percent of the total mental health care workforce in the health sector.

## Caregivers

Caregivers are formal employees in social welfare facilities. Each caregiver in the psychiatric care and rehabilitation centers can take care of two to 10 individuals with SMIs, depending on their psychiatric conditions. Caregivers are predominantly women between ages 26 and 45 whose educational attainment is mostly at the undergraduate level in various professions (Nguyen 2019).

Caregivers in psychiatric care and rehabilitation centers face numerous challenges in their daily work. Most of them reported difficulties in the early detection, prevention, classification, and counseling of mental disorders due to a lack of professional training and tools (HUPH 2019). Despite working hard in a challenging environment, the income for caregivers for people with SMIs is low, making it difficult to attract skilled employees to do this job (Viet Nam MOLISA 2021).

## Social collaborators

A hundred thousand lay social workers, known as social collaborators, serve in the national program on community-based social assistance for people with mental disorders. Lay social workers are often trusted community members playing a role in social organizations such as the Red Cross Union, Elderly Union, Youth's Union, Women's Union, Farmers' Union, Veterans Union, and others. Many perform multiple functions at the community level and may also function as village health workers. There is substantial variation in their training background, occupations, and experience (Chau et al. 2021).

In several provinces, the participation of social collaborators in community-based, task-sharing models has implications for improving the availability of and access to mental health care. By delivering low-cost depression care in rural communities, trained collaborators could fill a critical gap in care for mild to moderate depression, decrease depression symptoms among adults, increase mental health awareness and help-seeking in families, and reduce social marginalization and stigma in communities (Chau et al. 2021; Do, Nguyen, and Tran 2022; Murphy et al. 2020). Mental health support group intervention for people with SMIs, delivered by members of the Women's Union, provides promising evidence for addressing the mental health gap with high acceptability and feasibility (Nguyen et al. 2020).

However, there are policy-level challenges to the sustainable integration of social collaborators into the mental health systems. The social collaborators' scope of work in mental health care is undefined and unregulated. The lack of a professional development program for social collaborators can impact the quality of care and lead to professional demotivation. Furthermore, social collaborators are compensated incommensurately with their multiple responsibilities. The monthly allowance for a commune-level social collaborator is equivalent to the minimum salary level (from 3,250,000 VND to 4,680,000 VND, or from US$135 to US$195).[7] These factors may contribute to the high turnover rate of social collaborators (Chau et al. 2021).

## NOTES

1. Ministry of Education and Training Official Letter No. 9771/BGDĐT–HSSV, dated October 28, 2005, guided the implementation of counseling for students.
2. Prime Minister Decision No. 34/2020/QD-TTg, dated November 26, 2020, introduced a classification list of occupations in Viet Nam.
3. Ministry of Education and Training Circular No. 31/2017/TT-BGDĐT, dated December 18, 2017, provided guidance on psychology counseling for students in schools.
4. Ministry of Education and Training Official Letter No. 4252/BGDĐT-GDCTHSSV, dated August 31, 2022, guided psychological support counseling for students.
5. Ministry of Education and Training Official Letter No. 4252/BGDĐT-GDCTHSSV, dated August 31, 2022, guided psychological support and counseling for students.
6. Ministry of Labour, Invalids, and Social Affairs Circular 33/2017/TT-BLĐTBXH, dated December 29, 2017, provided guidance on organizational structure, staffing quota, social work procedures, and standards in social assistance facilities. Ministry of Labour, Invalids, and Social Affairs Circular 26/2022/TT-BLĐTBXH, dated December 12, 2022, regulated the codes, job title standards, and salary scale of social work officials.
7. Ministry of Labour, Invalids, and Social Affairs Circular 07/2013/TT-BLĐTBXH, dated May 4, 2013, regulated the professional qualifications of commune-level social collaborators.

## REFERENCES

Chau, L. W., J. Murphy, V. C. Nguyen, H. Lou, H. Khanh, T. Thu, H. Minas, and J. O'Neil. 2021. "Lay Social Workers Implementing a Task-Sharing Approach to Managing Depression in Vietnam." *International Journal of Mental Health Systems* 15: article 52. https://doi.org /10.1186/s13033-021-00478-8.

Do, M. T., T. T. Nguyen, and H. T. T. Tran. 2022. "Preliminary Results of Adapting the Stepped Care Model for Depression Management in Vietnam." *Frontiers in Psychiatry* 13: 922911. https://doi.org/10.3389/fpsyt.2022.922911.

HUPH (Hanoi University of Public Health). 2019. *Report on Social Work Systems in Hospitals.* Hanoi, Viet Nam: HUPH.

Le, H. D., M.-L. Nguyen-Thi, L. K. Tran, and T.-T. Tran-Thi. 2021. "Competency Framework of School Psychologists in Vietnam Schools." *International Journal of Ayurvedic Medicine* 12 (4): 897–901. https://doi.org/10.47552/ijam.v12i4.2118.

Murphy, J. K., H. Xie, V. C. Nguyen, L. W. Chau, P. T. Oanh, T. K. Nhu, J. O'Neil, et al. 2020. "Is Supported Self-Management for Depression Effective for Adults in Community-Based Settings in Vietnam? A Modified Stepped-Wedge Cluster Randomized Controlled Trial." *International Journal of Mental Health Systems* 14 (8). https://doi.org/10.1186 /s13033-020-00342-1.

Nguyen, T., T. Tran, S. Green, A. Hsueh, T. Tran, H. Tran, and J. Fisher. 2020. "Proof of Concept of Participant Informed, Psycho-Educational, Community-Based Intervention for People with Severe Mental Illness in Rural Vietnam." *International Journal of Social Psychiatry* 66 (3): 232–39. https://doi.org/10.1177/0020764019898234.

Nguyen, T. H. 2019. "Assessing Human Resources for Caring for People with Mental Disorders in Facilities Belonging to the Ministry of Labour, Invalids and Social Affairs." *Journal of Humanity and Social Sciences* 5 (6): 739–50.

Nguyen, T. M. H., V. S. Huynh, T. D. M. Nguyen, and V. L. Sam. 2018. "Solutions to Developing the School Counseling Staff in Vietnam." *Ho Chi Minh City University of Education Journal of Science, Education Science* 15 (10): 5–16.

Pham, A. K. 2021. *Introduction to Professional School Counseling in Vietnam.* India: Exceller Books.

Ta, T. M. T., K. Böge, T. D. Cao, G. Schomerus, T. D. Nguyen, M. Dettling, A. Mungee, et al. 2018. "Public Attitudes towards Psychiatrists in the Metropolitan Area of Hanoi, Vietnam." *Asian Journal of Psychiatry* 32: 44–49. https://doi.org/10.1016/j.ajp.2017.11.031.

Viet Nam MOH and MOET (Ministry of Health and Ministry of Education and Training of Viet Nam). 2017. *Report on Current State of School Health and Proposed Model in Vietnam.* Hanoi: Viet Nam MOH and MOET.

Viet Nam MOLISA (Ministry of Labour, Invalids, and Social Affairs of Viet Nam). 2021. *Draft Master Plan for the Social Welfare Network in the Period of 2021–2030 with a Vision to 2050.* Hanoi: Viet Nam MOLISA.

WHO (World Health Organization). 2021. *Mental Health Atlas 2020.* Geneva: WHO.

WHO and Viet Nam MOH (World Health Organization and Ministry of Health of Viet Nam). 2006. *WHO-AIMS Report on Mental Health System in Vietnam.* Geneva: WHO.

# 4 Mental Health Education and Training in Viet Nam

## INTRODUCTION

This chapter describes Viet Nam's education and training for psychiatry, mental health nursing, psychology, and social work. The chapter also identifies and analyzes constraints to the future development of the mental health workforce from the supply side.

## EDUCATION AND TRAINING FOR PSYCHIATRY

Career pathways and education frameworks in psychiatry have been established for decades, but competency requirements for psychiatrists are yet to be defined. Medical students take courses and clerkships in psychiatry through the undergraduate education program. General doctors and mental health doctors can become psychiatrists by completing a level 1 specialist program, a master's program, or a residency program. Some psychiatrists elect to study for additional years to earn a doctor of philosophy (PhD) degree or level 2 specialist degree (figure 4.1). However, there is neither a competency standard nor a competency examination for psychiatrists. General doctors can obtain a license to practice psychiatry upon completion of an 18-month internship in a psychiatric hospital.

Only one-third of the medical schools in Viet Nam offer a postgraduate education program in psychiatry, supplying nearly 100 new psychiatrists per year. As of 2021, Viet Nam had 27 medical schools, of which eight offered the level 1 specialist program; five, the level 2 specialist program; four, the master's degree program; three, the residency program; and three, the PhD program in psychiatry (figure 4.2). The three largest medical schools—Hanoi Medical University in the Northern region, Hue University of Medicine and Pharmacy in the Central region, and Ho Chi Minh City University of Medicine and Pharmacy in the Southern region—offer all the postgraduate programs. The common features of medical schools with postgraduate programs in psychiatry are a source of faculty lectures and a close link with major psychiatric hospitals in the area. However, the demand for specialization in psychiatry among general doctors

FIGURE 4.1

**Career pathway in psychiatry in Viet Nam**

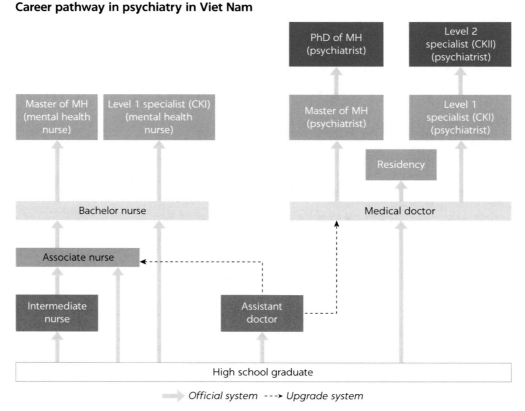

Source: Original figure for this report.
Note: CKI = first level specialization/specialist; CKII = second level specialization/specialist; MH = mental health.

FIGURE 4.2

**Psychiatry programs offered by medical universities in Viet Nam, 2021**

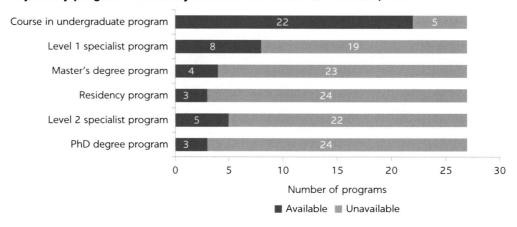

Source: Original figure for this report.
Note: "Unavailable" refers to the number of medical schools that do not offer the program.

remains low, mostly due to unfavorable working conditions. During 2016–20, only 100 general doctors enrolled in postgraduate psychiatry programs annually, which was a small supply for a country with a population of 100 million.

The country's programs are not yet fully aligned with competency-based education for psychiatrists. The curricula are over-prescriptive and focused on lectures. Case-based learning has been adopted in half of the courses, and simulation-based learning and role-playing are the most utilized methods of learning. Only one medical school offers an e-learning course. The undergraduate curricula present additional shortcomings. Although a few educational institutions, such as Hanoi Medical University, have updated their curricula to be more innovative and taught over a longer period, most of the training institutions still offer traditional education programs. They tend to consider mental health as a single specialty, which is learned in one session of two to three weeks, including theory and practice, in the fifth year of university. In addition to the duration, the content of the programs differs across training institutions and does not follow a standard framework. This leads to students losing interest in mental health majors.

In addition to the out-of-date curriculum, the shortage of resources for education in psychiatry poses a great challenge. At almost all the medical schools, the number of visiting lecturers is greater than the number of full-time faculty members. Five of the medical schools do not even have a single lecturer to run a psychiatry course, and six of the medical schools cannot employ a full-time lecturer in psychiatry. In the remaining medical schools, most of the lecturers are psychiatrists, 15 are associate professors, and only one is a full professor. Thirteen psychologists are employed in seven medical schools. Additionally, although there is a network of affiliated institutions for student practice, it is often overloaded due to too many students from different training programs. Some student practice institutions are too far from the training institution, making it difficult for students to arrange theoretical and practical learning time. Facilities and equipment for students to practice providing mental health care are also insufficient to meet the needs of the number of students.

Recently, psychiatry faculties have offered certification (nondegree) training courses in response to the increasing demand for continuing medical education (CME). Nine of 22 medical schools offer a psychiatry orientation training program, which is a six- or nine-month course. Over the past five years, the orientation training programs have equipped nearly 200 general doctors with basic knowledge and skills in psychiatry and enabled them to practice at the basic level upon completing the course. A few of the medical schools offer in-depth programs on schizophrenia and psychotic disorders (six months), child and adolescent psychiatry (three months), geriatric psychiatry (two months), stress-related disorders (two months), substance addiction (one month), and others (figure 4.3). So far, only Pham Ngoc Thach University has delivered a training program in clinical psychology (two weeks) and psychiatry in primary health care (one month), which need to be promoted and advanced toward achieving universal health coverage. Additionally, only one medical school has organized an online training program.

The government has implemented policies to encourage and attract people to study psychiatry. Compared to other specialties, psychiatry is one of the less attractive medical disciplines for people to research and practice. Therefore, based on the updated Law on Medical Examination and Treatment in 2023, from 2024, the government will support psychiatry majors by covering their tuition fees and living expenses during their studies. Specifically, for individuals studying at a state training institution in the health sector, 100 percent of their tuition fees and living expenses will be covered throughout the course. Although the government will not cover 100 percent of the tuition fees for students at private training institutions in the health sector, it will support them at a level corresponding to the level of support for students at state training institutions.

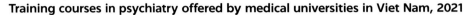

**FIGURE 4.3**

**Training courses in psychiatry offered by medical universities in Viet Nam, 2021**

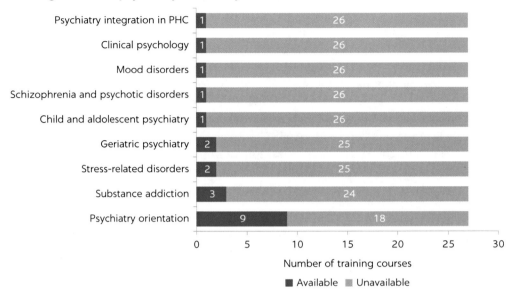

*Source:* Original figure for this report.
*Note:* "Unavailable" refers to the number of medical schools that do not offer the program. PHC = primary health care.

## EDUCATION AND TRAINING FOR MENTAL HEALTH NURSING

In Viet Nam, training for the nursing profession is carried out in various ways, from general to specialty nursing and from low to high levels of nursing education. According to the latest statistics from the Department of Science, Technology, and Training in the Ministry of Health, as of 2020, Viet Nam had about 38 nursing training institutions at the intermediate level, 83 at the college level, and 35 at the university level (table 4.1). According to 2020 data from the Viet Nam Nurses Association, annual targets included training about 5,700 intermediate trainees, 5,500 college students, and nearly 16,000 university students. In 2021, there were 17,996 graduating students and 54,857 students in training at the intermediate to tertiary levels. For postgraduate training, the country has four specialized nursing training institutions (including psychiatry), nine nursing training institutions at the master's level (five public and four privately funded), and only one nursing training institution at the doctoral level (Nam Dinh University of Nursing). The average total graduate enrollment target per year is more than 800 students. In 2021, 530 students graduated from doctoral, master's, and specialty-level programs, and 1,029 students were working toward graduating in the following years.

The mental health nursing curriculum is out of date and not harmonized across training institutions. The curriculum used by most training institutions was designed in 2001 at the latest, and the content sections need to be updated. Some up-to-date documents developed by large, reputable training institutions have yet to be published or officially taught.

To meet the demand for high-quality nursing services, Hanoi Medical University has developed an advanced practice nursing program. The program was designed based on the curriculum framework of the University of California, Long Beach, in the United States. It is a modern curriculum framework for training human nursing resources and meeting international standards at domestic and

**TABLE 4.1 Education institutions for health professionals in Viet Nam, 2020**

| DEGREES AND PROFESSIONS | PUBLIC SECTOR | | PRIVATE SECTOR | |
|---|---|---|---|---|
| | NUMBER OF INSTITUTIONS | PERCENTAGE OF TOTAL | NUMBER OF INSTITUTIONS | PERCENTAGE OF TOTAL |
| **Undergraduate degrees** | **21** | **42.9** | **28** | **57.1** |
| - Physicians | 18 | 66.7 | 9 | 33.3 |
| - Nurses | 14 | 40.0 | 21 | 60.0 |
| - Pharmacists | 16 | 43.2 | 21 | 56.8 |
| **Associate degrees** | **57** | **58.2** | **41** | **41.8** |
| - Nurses | 46 | 55.4 | 37 | 44.6 |
| - Pharmacists | 47 | 56.6 | 36 | 43.4 |
| **Intermediate degrees** | **10** | **26.3** | **28** | **73.7** |
| **TOTAL** | **88** | **47.5** | **97** | **52.5** |

*Source:* Ministry of Health of Viet Nam.

foreign medical institutions. In regular undergraduate nursing programs, students take classes on mental health for about 2 or 3 credits (including theory and practice). In the advanced practice nursing program, students are trained for up to 6 credits (3 theoretical and 3 practical). Thus, this will be a potential training program for developing nurses who are specialized in mental health in the future.

Psychiatric nurses are trained only at the postgraduate level. In Viet Nam, the mental health module of the undergraduate nursing education program is taught for a limited duration, for only 1 to 3 credits. There is a need for greater opportunities for graduate nurses to learn to practice competently in the mental health field. Therefore, several nursing education institutions have recently offered graduate education programs, including degrees for level 1 nurse specialists and masters of nursing in mental health. Only Nam Dinh Nursing University offers a doctorate program in psychiatric nursing; however, it has not yet had any graduates. Although more than 500 students are working toward master's and doctoral degrees in nursing annually, the number of those degrees in psychiatric nursing is minimal. Indeed, at the academic level, there is only one person with a PhD in psychiatric nursing, and that individual was trained in Taiwan, China. The lack of mental health nursing lecturers with postgraduate degrees hinders the development and operation of graduate mental health nursing education programs.

Mental health nurses receive ongoing training through CME classes on various topics. In addition to formal postgraduate psychiatric nursing training, to serve the urgent needs of society, training institutions have also developed and implemented short-term psychiatric nursing training programs. These programs are for one to three months for nurses working at mental health treatment facilities in the country. Most of the nursing training institutions with mental health departments hold CME classes, and psychiatric nurses may receive private continuing training or joint training with psychiatrists. Some training institutions have engaged in international cooperation activities, inviting mental health professionals from abroad to organize continuing training courses to disseminate and update new knowledge for psychiatric doctors and nurses. However, the rate of ongoing training in mental health for nurses is much lower than that for doctors. A study conducted at 10 mental health hospitals showed that although the nursing workforce is three to four times larger than that of doctors, the proportion of nurses with CME certification is less than 1 percent. In contrast, among doctors, it is over 20 percent.

## EDUCATION AND TRAINING FOR PSYCHOLOGY

As of 2023, 32 universities in Viet Nam were running a psychology education program. Most of the psychology education programs offer degrees at the bachelor's level, six offer master's level degrees, and five offer degrees at the doctoral level. The areas of study include general psychology, school psychology, educational psychology, clinical psychology, social psychology, and industrial-organizational psychology. Traditional programs for providing psychology education are no longer predominant. Instead, new graduate programs have appeared, in which clinical psychology and school psychology are two recently emerging trends (Sirikantraporn, Nguyen, and Hoang 2020).

Many psychology education institutions are concentrated in the Red River Delta and Southeast regions. Specialized programs in clinical psychology are found only in Hanoi and Ho Chi Minh City. Given the unequal distribution of psychology education institutions, there is substantial geographic variation in access to psychology education programs.

Several collaborative programs between Viet Nam and foreign universities have been created in clinical psychology. For example, the master's degree in clinical psychology was developed between Hanoi University of Humanities and Social Science and Toulouse Le Mirail University (in France). The master's degree in child and adolescent clinical psychology was designed between Hanoi University of Education and Vanderbilt University (in the United States). A recent movement in the field has been the expansion of applied psychology, with foreign support for establishing supervisory practices for new practitioners, conducting psychology research, developing networking, and building new practicum sites for psychology students to learn the needed skills. For instance, circa 2004–05, experts from the Ecole des psychologues Practiciens de Paris collaborated with local professionals to create clinical psychology class units at the Ho Chi Minh City Pediatric Hospital No. 1 and No. 2 (Sirikantraporn, Nguyen, and Hoang 2020).

Despite recent developments, psychology education in Viet Nam still needs to overcome various challenges. For example, there is no competency framework for psychologists to guide faculties in designing education programs. The curricula are over-prescriptive, focused on lectures, and should be adaptable to new educational priorities. The resources for psychology education are insufficient in various aspects, including human resources, teaching infrastructure, and learning materials. The lack of standardized practice sites and qualified preceptors poses significant challenges for students in clinical psychology to develop clinical and ethical competencies. The career paths of students from psychology programs often need to be clarified and expanded. Registration and licensing systems for psychologists, including clinical psychologists, have yet to be established, which affects graduates' employability and professional promotion. Thus, there is an urgent need to strengthen the governance framework and enhance the quality of education and training in clinical psychology.

## EDUCATION AND TRAINING FOR SOCIAL WORK

In Viet Nam, social work education and training include higher education, vocational training, and short-term training. Those who wish to pursue this career can choose a full-time study program with increasing levels of education, with degrees at the intermediate, college, bachelor's, master's, and doctoral levels.

Those who want to improve their capacity to provide social assistance to people with mental disorders can attend short-term training programs.

## Higher education and vocational training for social work

The country has 55 higher education institutions and 21 vocational training institutions for social work, which supply about 6,500 individuals to the labor market yearly (Nguyen 2022). Among the higher education institutions, 50 have bachelor's degree programs, 20 have master's degree programs, and two have doctorate programs (Nguyen 2023). However, the higher education institutions for social work are unevenly distributed and concentrated mainly in the Red River Delta and Mekong Delta regions. Only six higher education institutions are scattered across the mountainous areas of the North, Central, and Central Highlands regions.

The mental health modules in social work education and training programs are inconsistent. Because there are no competency standards for social workers, schools define the learning outcomes and develop resource-oriented frameworks. Most vocational and higher education programs for social work only introduce students to the basics, rather than providing practical skills training in mental health care. Recently, Hanoi University of Public Health offered its first undergraduate program for social work in health. The program's training modules that are directly related to psychology and mental health account for 8 credits (table 4.2).

Resources for teaching and learning are limited, especially in specialized areas of mental health. Due to the small number of training institutions and targets for training students working on master's and doctoral degrees in social work, lecturers teaching about social work are lacking in both quantity and quality, especially in specialized fields such as mental health care. Although the Ministry of Labour, Invalids, and Social Affairs has directly organized dozens of training courses for trainers on mental health care for localities every year, it has been unable to meet all the training needs. The basic curriculum is complete, but most of the subjects are basic, and there are no specialized materials. Some documents are still at the rough translation level and need to be customized to fit the social situation in Viet Nam.

The network of social work practice facilities for mental health care is also a barrier to training. Given the rapid expansion of social work education, universities in Viet Nam face tremendous challenges in organizing effective field practicums, including a lack of qualified field supervisors, inadequate student assessment

**TABLE 4.2 Mental health content in social work training programs**

| UNDERGRADUATE PROGRAMS | | POSTGRADUATE PROGRAMS |
|---|---|---|
| **HEALTH SECTOR ORIENTATION** | **SOCIAL SECTOR ORIENTATION** | |
| Basic health science modules | Basic behavioral science modules | Advanced behavioral science modules |
| Basic psychology and clinical psychology modules | Social work in the mental health care module | Behavioral health in social work modules |
| Social and health rehabilitation modules | Consultation and basic counseling practice | Applied consultation in the intervention of specific target groups in social work |
| Social work in the mental health care module | | Intervention with specific groups, including those with mental disorders |
| Social work practices with individuals, groups, and in the community | | Studies on mental health in social work for specific groups |

*Sources:* Original table for this report; Nguyen 2023.

methods, and loose collaboration between universities and field agencies (Cohen et al. 2019), particularly clinical practice sites for mental health care.

### Short-term training for social work in mental health care

In parallel with the formal training programs, short-term continuing training programs are organized to improve the quality of social work services. Specifically, in mental health care, the Department of Social Protection has cooperated with the University of Labor and Social Affairs and social work training institutions to develop a methodical, short-term training program for social work (box 4.1). According to statistics from the University of Labor and Social Affairs, from 2013 to 2022, more than 10 short-term, 33-day courses on mental health care were held in three regions in the North, Central, and South, with more than 1,000 trainees. Experienced lecturers from Viet Nam and abroad participated in these courses.

### Training for social work for collaborators and community workers

There are competency standards for training social work collaborators. Specifically, they need to understand the process and skills for practicing social work at a basic level to support the subject as well as the policy regime. Additionally, they are expected to acknowledge the responsibilities and duties of a social work collaborator to perform effective coordination with relevant stakeholders on social work tasks. Social work collaborators are required to have a certificate for participating in short-term training on social work, or an educational background that is suitable for social work tasks, such as psychology, sociology, special education, or other related studies. Social work collaborators must also have a good moral character with no criminal record.

Short-term training courses are regularly organized for social work collaborators. At the local level, social work centers coordinate with social work training schools to organize training courses to improve the professional and social work skills of social work collaborators. These training programs usually take place

---

**Box 4.1**

### Social work training for mental health care

1. Laws and policies for the development of the social work profession
2. Mental health care fundamentals
3. Clinical psychology
4. Mental health awareness–raising communication
5. Care and rehabilitation for some forms of mental illness
6. Treatment for patients with mental illness
7. Social work in mental health care
8. Basic consultation in mental health care
9. Shift management in psychiatric care and rehabilitation

*Source:* Nguyen (2023).

over two to three days, and the classes have about 100 students. The training includes communication issues on community-based social work programs and guidance on methods of care and management of subjects such as children, people with mental illnesses, and others.

There is still insufficient training because of financial issues. Because the social work collaborator position is frequently rotated, retraining must be implemented for the new personnel. However, in many communes, especially in remote areas, the authorities find it difficult to manage the budget. In some cases, the previous collaborators must instruct the new ones; however, there will be no certificate and this situation cannot ensure the quality of the training outcome.

## REFERENCES

Cohen E., A. Hines, L. Drabble, H. Nguyen, M. Han, S. Sen, and D. Faires. 2019. *The International Development of Social Work Education: The Vietnam Experience*. Abingdon: Routledge.

Nguyen, C. T. 2022. "Development of Social Work in Viet Nam and Orientation in the Period of 2021–2030." Paper presented at the Workshop on Policy and Legal Framework for Social Work in the Justice Sector, Central Committee of Propaganda and Education, e-Newspaper of the Viet Nam Communist Party, Ministry of Labor, Invalids, and Social Affairs, Hanoi, December 1.

Nguyen, T. H. 2023. "Education and Training Programs on Social Work in Mental Healthcare in Viet Nam." Paper presented at the Workshop on Mental Health Education in Viet Nam, Hanoi Medical University, GIZ, and World Bank, Hanoi, March 23.

Sirikantraporn, S., H. A. Nguyen, and T.-H. L. Hoang. 2020. "Teaching Psychology in Vietnam." In *Teaching Psychology around the World*, volume 5, edited by G. J. Rich, A. Padilla López, L. Ebersöhn, J. Taylor, and S. Morrissey, 384–99. Cambridge Scholars Publisher.

# 5 Conclusions and Recommendations

## CONCLUSIONS

The population coverage of mental health services in Viet Nam has improved through four interconnected domains: health care, social welfare, education, and informal systems. The numbers of psychiatric beds in hospitals and social protection centers have increased steadily, and networks of community-based health and social work facilities have expanded at a rapid pace. Although institutional care remains dominant, community-based programs have been implemented in the health and social sectors. The education sector in Viet Nam has made progress in addressing the mental health needs of children and adolescents by introducing inclusive education policies and setting guidelines for school-based mental health services. In addition to formal care, informal mental health services are available, and they are vital for providing care to people with mental disorders. Additionally, the growth of social networks and online communities has led to the rise of peer support groups.

Nevertheless, the mental health systems in Viet Nam still face systematic problems and structural challenges. The uneven distribution of psychiatric services leads to unequal access across the provinces and an urban-rural divide. The dominance of traditional treatment regimens in many psychiatric hospitals restricts the adoption of an evidence-based combination of nonpharmacological interventions, such as psychotherapies and psychosocial rehabilitation. The shortage of resources hinders mental health care service providers from reaching and maintaining the quality of care required to meet the basic needs of people with mental disorders and support them toward recovery. Although the government has gradually transitioned to community-based care and achieved some progress in this direction, obstacles remain that need to be addressed.

The mental health workforce presents a major challenge facing the mental health care system's ability to achieve universal mental health coverage. Despite recent developments in all professions, the quantity and quality of the mental health workforce have yet to meet the demand. Almost all the human resources for mental health care in Viet Nam are still below the global average in education and numbers. The distribution of the workforce is uneven and mainly concentrated in advantaged and wealthier areas, leading to disparities in access to mental health care. Because of the lack of standardized training, certification, and qualification processes, a majority of the staff in the field of psychiatry have yet to undergo formal psychiatric training. There is high job dissatisfaction among employees working in the mental health field, with their primary concerns being about income and fringe benefits. Furthermore, due to budget constraints, institutions find it difficult to retain qualified staff.

Viet Nam has numerous training and education institutions at various levels, with a considerable number of students graduating every year. However, psychiatric training at the university level is limited and primarily conducted at the postgraduate level, with fewer graduates specializing in mental health care. Moreover, the psychiatric training programs are inconsistent across institutions due to the lack of professional standards. Training resources, including lecturers and infrastructure, could be improved, and many training materials need to be updated to be appropriate for the current demand. Additionally, although continuing medical education programs are available, only some staff members are sent to be trained.

## RECOMMENDATIONS

A national strategic plan should be developed to align mental health workforce development with employer demands and population needs. The key stakeholders include government agencies (the Ministry of Health, the Ministry of Education and Training, the Ministry of Labour, Invalids, and Social Affairs, and the Provincial People Committees), mental health facilities, professional associations, and the academic community. These stakeholders should work together to analyze the situation, set priorities and targets, and harmonize the supply and demand for mental health professionals to meet the needs of the population and the challenges facing the health system. This joint planning exercise requires shared data across stakeholders, strengthened multisectoral and multiprofessional coordination, as well as improved institutional capacity to make mental health workforce projections for future needs and conduct evidence-based decision-making (Australia 2022; Funk and Drew 2015; WHO 2005). In the planning process, special attention should be paid to the systematic problems of the mental health workforce, including the shortage of workers, competency mismatch, skill mix imbalance, maldistribution, and weak workforce governance framework. The ultimate purpose is to ensure a sufficient, competent, and well-coordinated mental health workforce toward achieving universal coverage of mental health services.

The development of a sufficient and competent mental health workforce requires substantial changes in the education and training systems. Mental health education institutions need to balance the criteria for admissions with professional and geographic shortages, develop and adopt competency-based curricula that are responsive to changing needs, expand education programs to a wider scope of professions and degrees, promote interprofessional education to enhance team-based care, strengthen resources for education with emphasis on faculty development, and adopt digital technology. To offer students adequate practical experience, mental health education institutions must expand their networks of practice sites beyond traditional psychiatric hospitals to outpatient clinics and community-based mental health care settings, ensure that the necessary resources are provided for clinical instruction, and improve supervision of practice. To expand access to in-service training and continuous professional development, it is recommended that mental health training institutions should advance e-learning courses in addition to onsite classroom instruction. E-learning courses have proved effective in closing competency gaps in the existing mental health workforce, especially for those who serve in remote areas. The pursuit of such reforms will require institutional and instructional changes as well as intensive investment in health professional education and training systems from all sources, including public, private, and international aid (Le 2017, 2021a, 2021b, 2023; World Bank 2022).

The available mental health workforce should be distributed equitably and sustainably, be fit for purpose, and be responsive to most needs. A priority area is the recruitment, deployment, and retention of mental health professionals for disadvantaged provinces, particularly those in the Northern Upland, Central Highlands, and Southwest regions, to close the urban-rural divide in mental health coverage. Mechanisms for attracting and retaining the health workforce in rural areas, such as the "Health Professional Rotation from the Upper Level to the Lower Level" program[1] and the "Young Volunteer Doctors for Remote Areas" program,[2] should be expanded to the mental health professions. In addition to improving mental health workers' fringe benefits and rewards, more effort should be made to harmonize operating rules and procedures within mental health facilities. These have been identified as critical areas of job dissatisfaction among mental health professionals. At the grassroots level, technology-enabled models (counseling hotlines, teleconsultation, and others) and collaborative task-shifting and -sharing models, in which mental health care is shifted from specialized professionals to nonspecialized practitioners, should be scaled up to improve access to integrated mental health care in settings with limited resources.[3] It is also advised that mental health managers should develop further competencies related to human resource management.

A workforce governance framework is pivotal for creating a conducive environment for mental health professionals. This entails standardization and regulation as well as registration and licensure. Relevant professional associations should define the competency standards for the mental health professions, paving the way for competency-based education, licensing examination, recruitment, and pay. The Ministry of Health, in collaboration with the Ministry of Labour, Invalids, and Social Affairs, the Ministry of Education and Training, and professional associations, should determine the scope of practices and code of ethics that mental health workers are permitted to perform, particularly in emerging areas such as clinical psychology, school psychology, and social work. The National Medical Council should make intensive efforts to develop guidelines, blueprints, question banks, examiners, and information systems to realize the legal requirements for licensing examinations for the mental health professions. While licensure is legally required for clinical practitioners, registration should be a regulatory requirement for psychological counselors and mental health social workers as well. These activities should be implemented under the leadership of a (self-) governing body, such as a mental health professions council, with mandates to set standards for education and practices, keep a register of professionals, and conduct competency examinations for licensure.

Financing is a powerful tool for transforming the mental health workforce toward achieving the goal of universal health coverage. Mental health policy makers and managers can start by mapping the current resources to understand the reasons why the mental health workforce has been underfunded for so long.

The resource base for the mental health workforce may be developed through investment projects or financial mechanisms, such as the establishment of an innovation fund to strengthen the mental health workforce, expanded public insurance coverage of primary mental health care services, increased incentive packages for skilled professionals in rural areas, and others. Taking efficiency and effectiveness into account, mental health policy makers in Viet Nam should use these financial tools to incentivize mental health providers to integrate mental health into primary health care and shift from institutional care to community-based care.[4] It is important to allocate resources to the priorities set forth by the national strategic plan for development of the mental health workforce. To narrow the urban-rural divide and regional disparities in mental health coverage, special attention should be paid to attracting and retaining skilled professionals in underserved areas, particularly in the Central Highlands and Northern Upland regions.

## NOTES

1. Viet Nam's health sector has been implementing the "Health Professional Rotation from the Upper Level to the Lower Level" program since 2008 under Ministry of Health Decision 1816/QĐ-BYT, dated May 26, 2028. The program's objectives are to improve the quality of care and train health professionals at the lower level, particularly for health facilities in remote areas. Between 2008 and 2018, more than 10,000 health professionals at central-level facilities were rotated and transferred more than 5,400 medical techniques to provincial-level facilities; 3,800 health professionals at provincial-level facilities were rotated and transferred 3,500 medical techniques to district-level facilities; and 3,800 health professionals at district-level facilities were rotated and transferred 1,900 medical techniques to commune health stations.

2. Viet Nam's health sector has been implementing the "Young Volunteer Doctors for Remote Areas" program since 2013 under Ministry of Health Decision 585/QĐ-BYT, dated February 20, 2013. The program's objective is to supply specialized doctors to the most disadvantaged districts. Between 2013 and 2021, 354 specialized doctors, of whom 78 percent were from ethnic minorities and 40 percent were female, were trained and dispatched to work in the poorest districts on a rotation basis (World Bank 2022).

3. The World Health Organization's Mental Health Gap Action Programme supports comprehensive, integrated, and responsive mental health and social care services delivered through community platforms. Community workers and health care providers who are affiliated with primary health care services can be trained in using scalable psychological interventions to bridge the gap in the availability of evidence-based psychological services (https://www.who.int/westernpacific/activities/developing-community -based-mental-health-services). In Viet Nam, collaborative task-shifting and -sharing models, in which mental care is shifted from specialized professionals to nonspecialized practitioners, have proved effective at the commune level. Viet Nam's Ministry of Labour, Invalids, and Social Affairs has been developing and scaling up community-based models for rehabilitation and social assistance for people with mental disorders.

4. High-income countries have been "deinstitutionalizing"—moving people out of psychiatric hospitals toward care in the community. In some countries, such as Italy, the United Kingdom, and the United States, the deinstitutionalization process started over 50 years ago (OECD 2014).

# REFERENCES

Australia. 2022. "National Mental Health Workforce Strategy 2022–2032: Executive Summary." Government of Australia, Canberra. https://www.health.gov.au/sites/default/files/2023 -06/national-mental-health-workforce-strategy-summary.pdf.

Funk, M. K., and N. J. Drew. 2015. "Mental Health Policy and Strategic Plan." *Eastern Mediterranean Health Journal* 21 (7): 522–26.

Le, S. M. 2017. "What Hinders Viet Nam's Path to Universal Healthcare? The Lack of Human Capital," *World Bank Blogs*, July 24, 2017. https://blogs.worldbank.org/eastasiapacific/what -hinders-vietnams-path-universal-healthcare-lack-human-capital.

Le, S. M. 2021a. "How Information Technology Is Improving Nursing Education in Viet Nam," World Bank Blogs, May 12, 2021. https://blogs.worldbank.org/eastasiapacific/how -information-technology-improving-nursing-education-vietnam.

Le, S. M. 2021b. "The Windy Journey of Medical Education in Viet Nam," World Bank Blogs, January 19, 2021. https://blogs.worldbank.org/health/windy-journey-medical-education -vietnam.

Le, S. M. 2023. "Building a Competent Workforce for Oral and Dental Care in ASEAN," World Bank Blogs, April 3, 2024. https://blogs.worldbank.org/en/eastasiapacific/building-a -competent-workforce-for-oral-and-dental-care-in-asean.

OECD (Organisation for Economic Co-operation and Development). 2014. *Making Mental Health Count: The Social and Economic Costs of Neglecting Mental Health Care.* Paris: OECD Publishing. https://www.oecd.org/els/health-systems/Focus-on-Health-Making-Mental -Health-Count.pdf.

WHO (World Health Organization). 2005. *The WHO Mental Health Policy and Service Guidance Package Module 8: Human Resources and Training in Mental Health.* Geneva: WHO.

World Bank. 2022. *Vietnam: Health Professionals Education and Training for Health System Reforms Project.* Washington, DC: World Bank Group.